TACHDJIAN'S
PROCEDURES
IN PEDIATRIC
ORTHOPAEDICS

from the Texas Scottish Rite
Hospital for Children

TACHDJIAN'S
PROCEDURES
IN PEDIATRIC
ORTHOPAEDICS

from the Texas Scottish Rite
Hospital for Children

John A. Herring, MD

Chief of Staff Emeritus
Texas Scottish Rite Hospital for Children
Professor of Orthopaedic Surgery
The University of Texas Southwestern Medical Center
Dallas, Texas

ELSEVIER

ELSEVIER

1600 John F. Kennedy Blvd.
Ste 1800
Philadelphia, PA 19103-2899

TACHDJIAN'S PROCEDURES IN PEDIATRIC ORTHOPAEDICS   ISBN: 978-0-323-44808-6

Notices

Knowledge and best practice in this field are constantly changing. As new research and experience
broaden our understanding, changes in research methods, professional practices, or medical
treatment may become necessary.

Practitioners and researchers must always rely on their own experience and knowledge in
evaluating and using any information, methods, compounds, or experiments described herein. In
using such information or methods they should be mindful of their own safety and the safety of
others, including parties for whom they have a professional responsibility.

With respect to any drug or pharmaceutical products identified, readers are advised to check the
most current information provided (i) on procedures featured or (ii) by the manufacturer of each
product to be administered, to verify the recommended dose or formula, the method and duration
of administration, and contraindications. It is the responsibility of practitioners, relying on their own
experience and knowledge of their patients, to make diagnoses, to determine dosages and the best
treatment for each individual patient, and to take all appropriate safety precautions.

To the fullest extent of the law, neither the Publisher nor the authors, contributors, or editors,
assume any liability for any injury and/or damage to persons or property as a matter of products
liability, negligence or otherwise, or from any use or operation of any methods, products,
instructions, or ideas contained in the material herein.

Library of Congress Cataloging-in-Publication Data

Names: Herring, John A., editor. | Texas Scottish Rite Hospital for Children.
Title: Tachdjian's procedures in pediatric orthopaedics : from the Texas
    Scottish Rite Hospital for Children / [edited by] John A. Herring.
Other titles: Procedures in pediatric orthopaedics
Description: Philadelphia, PA : Elsevier, [2017] | The procedures are from
    Tachdjian's Pediatric Orthopaedics, Fifth Edition. | Includes
    bibliographical references and index.
Identifiers: LCCN 2015045931 | ISBN 9780323448086 (hardcover : alk. paper)
Subjects: | MESH: Orthopedic Procedures | Child | Musculoskeletal
    Diseases–surgery
Classification: LCC RD732.3.C48 | NLM WS 270 | DDC 618.927–dc23 LC record available at
http://lccn.loc.gov/2015045931

International Standard Book Number: 978-0-323-44808-6

Content Strategist: Katy Meert
Publishing Services Manager: Catherine Jackson
Senior Project Manager: Rachel E. McMullen
Design Direction: Ashley Miner

Printed in Canada

Last digit is the print number: 9 8 7 6 5 4 3 2

Working together
to grow libraries in
developing countries

www.elsevier.com • www.bookaid.org

Contributors

Daniel J. Sucato, MD

Associate Editor
Chief of Staff
Texas Scottish Rite Hospital for Children;
Professor of Orthopaedic Surgery
The University of Texas Southwestern Medical Center;
Staff Orthopaedist
Children's Medical Center
Dallas, Texas

Mark C. Gebhardt, MD

Frederick W. and Jane Ilfed Professor of Orthopaedic
  Surgery
Harvard Medical School;
Chief of Orthoapedic Surgery
Beth Israel Deaconess Medical Center;
Associate in Orthopaedic Surgery
Children's Hospital Boston
Boston, Massachusetts

John A. Herring, MD

Chief of Staff Emeritus
Texas Scottish Rite Hospital for Children;
Professor of Orthopaedic Surgery
The University of Texas Southwestern Medical Center
Dallas, Texas

Christine Ho, MD

Staff Orthopaedist
Texas Scottish Rite Hospital for Children;
Assistant Professor of Orthopaedic Surgery
The University of Texas Southwestern Medical Center
Dallas, Texas

Charles E. Johnston, MD

Assistant Chief of Staff
Texas Scottish Rite Hospital for Children;
Professor of Orthopaedic Surgery
The University of Texas Southwestern Medical Center
Dallas, Texas

Lori A. Karol, MD

Staff Orthopaedist
Texas Scottish Rite Hospital for Children;
Professor of Orthopaedic Surgery
The University of Texas Southwestern Medical Center
Dallas, Texas

Karl E. Rathjen, MD

Staff Orthopaedist
Texas Scottish Rite Hospital for Children;
Professor
Department of Orthopaedic Surgery
The University of Texas Southwestern Medical Center;
Chief of Clinical Service
Department of Orthopaedic Surgery
Children's Medical Center
Dallas, Texas

Anthony I. Riccio, MD

Staff Orthopaedist
Texas Scottish Rite Hospital for Children;
Assistant Professor
Department of Orthopaedic Surgery
The University of Texas Southwestern Medical Center;
Staff Orthopaedist
Children's Medical Center
Dallas, Texas

B. Stephens Richards, MD

Chief Medical Officer
Texas Scottish Rite Hospital for Children;
Professor of Orthopaedic Surgery
The University of Texas Southwestern Medical Center
Dallas, Texas

Philip L. Wilson, MD

Staff Orthopaedist
Texas Scottish Rite Hospital for Children;
Associate Professor
Department of Orthopaedic Surgery
The University of Texas Southwestern Medical Center;
Staff Orthopaedist
Children's Medical Center
Dallas, Texas

Preface

Performing orthopedic surgery for children is a wonderfully fulfilling endeavor with great potential benefit for the child. It is also a difficult and challenging field as well, and poorly chosen or performed surgery may produce lasting harm. Children present with complex problems which frequently are unique and not found in textbooks. The child is growing and surgery must enhance and preserve growth whenever possible.

This text includes 69 common and rare surgical procedures in pediatric orthopaedics. The procedures are from *Tachdjian's Pediatric Orthopaedics, Fifth Edition*, organized into clear sections so readers can quickly find the procedure they are looking for. This is an ideal text for those new to the operating room who want a clear description of our recommended and preferred techniques; it's also perfect for those who have been practicing for some time but want a quick refresher before going into surgery or want to see alternative techniques.

The surgeon must carefully consider many factors before proceeding with surgery, including the question of his or her own experience and technical competence to do the needed operation. The surgeon must be open not only to second opinions, but should actively consult colleagues and authorities when the best course for the patient is not clear. It is imperative that parents and children participate fully in the decision making process as much as possible. Thus a monograph devoted to surgical techniques, by definition, leaves out the most important part of the process; the decision making part, the part where a surgery is chosen for a young person. The surgeon must understand the disease process, its natural history, its prognosis untreated verses the likely response to surgery. The understanding includes preoperative and postoperative planning, consideration of complications, and possible negative outcomes. All of this is covered in scientific publications and textbooks and cannot be considered in depth in this small book. Certainly we would recommend that the surgeon review the relevant chapters in the *Tachdjian's Pediatric Orthopaedics, Fifth Edition* text whenever needed.

We, the authors of this work, are more than well-qualified for the task. The Texas Scottish Rite Hospital for Children has been taking care of children with orthopedic problems since 1921. We currently have 19 full-time pediatric orthopedists on our staff. Our group meets twice weekly to discuss surgical indications, techniques, and outcomes of a very large number of surgeries. We continuously review and publish results of analyses of all aspects of our surgical and nonsurgical activities. From this base we are constantly considering new procedures, improving results with existing ones, while realizing that there is no standing still in an advancing medical science.

Our book is well illustrated and we believe that the procedures are well described. The reader is also encouraged to make use of the cases in our video library. These videos are live action recording of operations, carefully edited to present the relevant steps in an efficient manner. Many surgeons around the world have told us how much they value the videos which accompany *Tachdjian's Pediatric Orthopaedics, 5th Edition*, and which they often view while performing their surgeries.

Contents

SECTION V
UPPER EXTREMITY DISORDERS

VIDEO CONTENTS

SECTION I

HIP DISORDERS

Surgical intervention is often necessary for developmental dislocation of the hip. For those who are missed in the newborn period, and for those who fail early treatment with splinting, surgery is usually necessary. We prefer to perform closed reduction, with the possible need for open reduction, in children at least 6 months of age. A gentle closed reduction is performed under general anesthesia and if stable is confirmed with an arthrogram. When closed reduction fails, an open reduction is needed. The medial approach is best for children before one year of age, and an anterior open reduction is favored thereafter. The medial approach is done through a small incision, visualization can be difficult, and great care is required to avoid avascular necrosis. Children of walking age may require femoral shortening to safely reduce the hip, and children older than 18 months may also benefit from a Salter or Pemberton osteotomy. We do not find that femoral derotation procedures are beneficial in most cases.

In performing a varus osteotomy, we find that a mild amount of varus (10 to 15 degrees) is usually all that is required. The femoral shaft should be medially displaced with a varus osteotomy and laterally displaced with a valgus procedure.

For slipped capital epiphysis, a fully threaded screw, centrally placed to avoid joint penetration, provides excellent stabilization of the slip. The treatment of the unstable slip is controversial. Pinning in situ has a lower rate of avascular necrosis than reduction methods and may require subsequent corrective osteotomy. Open reduction requires very careful preservation of the retinacular vasculature, and success depends on the experience and advanced training of the surgeon.

Osteotomies for acetabular dysplasia include Salter and Pemberton for younger children, triple pelvic osteotomies in the late childhood to early adolescent group, and periacetabular surgery for nearly mature adolescents. The later procedures are also complex and require the surgeon to have advanced training.

Procedure 1   Closed Reduction and Casting for Developmental Dislocation of the Hip (see Video 1)

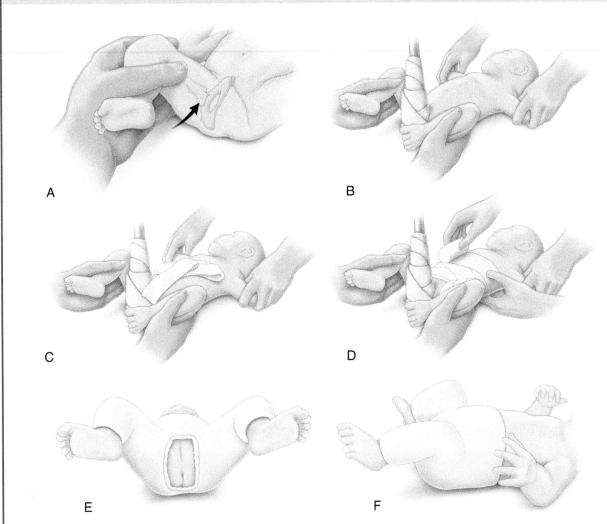

A, The first step of this procedure—evaluating the reduction of the hip—is probably the most important. With the infant completely anesthetized, the surgeon gently performs the Ortolani maneuver by grasping the infant's thigh, applying mild longitudinal traction, lifting the greater trochanter with the fingers, and abducting the hip to reduce the femoral head. The reduction should be done with the hip flexed approximately 120 degrees. After the patient's hip reduces, the surgeon evaluates its stability by extending the hip to the point of redislocation and then adducting the hip to the point of redislocation. A reduction is considered stable if the hip can be adducted 20 to 30 degrees from maximal abduction and extended to less than 90 degrees without redislocation. An arthrogram may be obtained at this time to further assess the adequacy of the reduction. If the adductors are tight on palpation with the hip in the reduced position, a tenotomy of the adductor longus may be performed to reduce pressure on the hip.

B, After the reduction is established, the patient is placed on the infant spica table for cast application. The head of the table is raised to assist with keeping the perineum against the center post. At this point, the surgeon should be certain of the reduction of the hip. He or she should hold the hips to maintain the reduction while avoiding extremes of abduction or internal rotation.

C, A rolled towel or stockinette is placed over the child's abdomen and later removed to allow for breathing room in the cast.

D, Cast padding is applied around the abdomen in a figure-eight pattern around the groin and then down the legs. The first cast is usually applied to the middle of the calf of the affected extremity and to above the knee on the contralateral leg. If available, a layer of moisture-control material (e.g., Gore-Tex) may be placed against the skin to prevent wetness. Casting material (usually fiberglass) is then rolled over the areas to be enclosed. During the entire procedure, the surgeon must continually assess the infant's hip position by abducting the hips maximally and then "backing off" by at least 15 degrees to prevent the hip from sagging into full abduction.

E, The infant is taken off of the table, and the cast is windowed for perineal access. Radiographs are obtained at this point to ensure reduction. If any doubt remains regarding reduction, minimal-cut computed tomography is useful to confirm the hip's position.

F, Side view of the finished cast.

Procedure 2   Medial Approach for Open Reduction of the Developmentally Dislocated Hip

The patient is placed supine, and the ipsilateral hip, the hemipelvis, and the entire lower limb are prepared and draped in the usual fashion, which allows for the free mobility of the limb during surgery.

We prefer a transverse skin incision because it affords better access to the hip and results in better cosmesis than a longitudinal incision. The hip is approached anterior to the pectineus with the traditional Ludloff technique. An alternative approach—posterior to the pectineus—is also described.

Transverse Skin Incision With Surgical Approach Anterior and Lateral to the Pectineus

A, The preferred approach is through a transverse oblique skin incision that is 5 to 7 cm long, centered over the anterior margin of the adductor longus, and approximately 1 cm distal and parallel to the inguinal crease.

The deep fascia is divided. The surgeon should be careful not to injure the saphenous vein; however, if necessary, the vein can be ligated and sectioned.

B and **C,** The hip is approached anterior to the pectineus, between that muscle and the femoral sheath. With this approach, the pectineus muscle is retracted medially and inferiorly and the femoral vessels and nerve are retracted laterally, thereby exposing the iliopsoas tendon as it passes toward the lesser trochanter. The femoral circumflex vessels cross the field and are carefully retracted laterally.

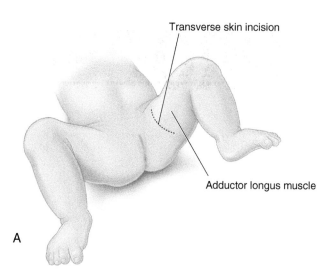

Transverse skin incision

Adductor longus muscle

A

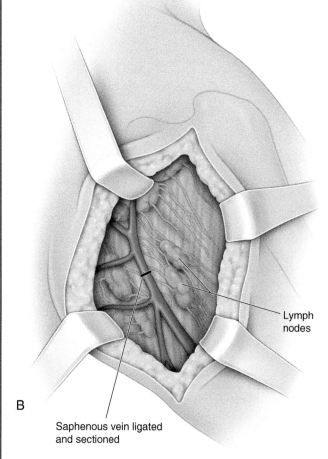

Lymph nodes

Saphenous vein ligated and sectioned

B

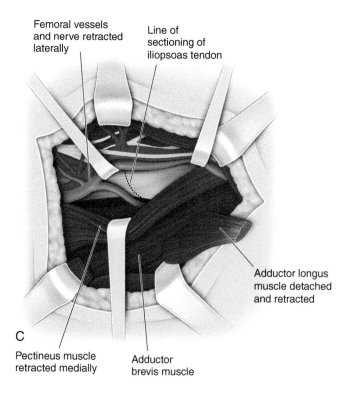

Femoral vessels and nerve retracted laterally

Line of sectioning of iliopsoas tendon

Adductor longus muscle detached and retracted

Pectineus muscle retracted medially

Adductor brevis muscle

C

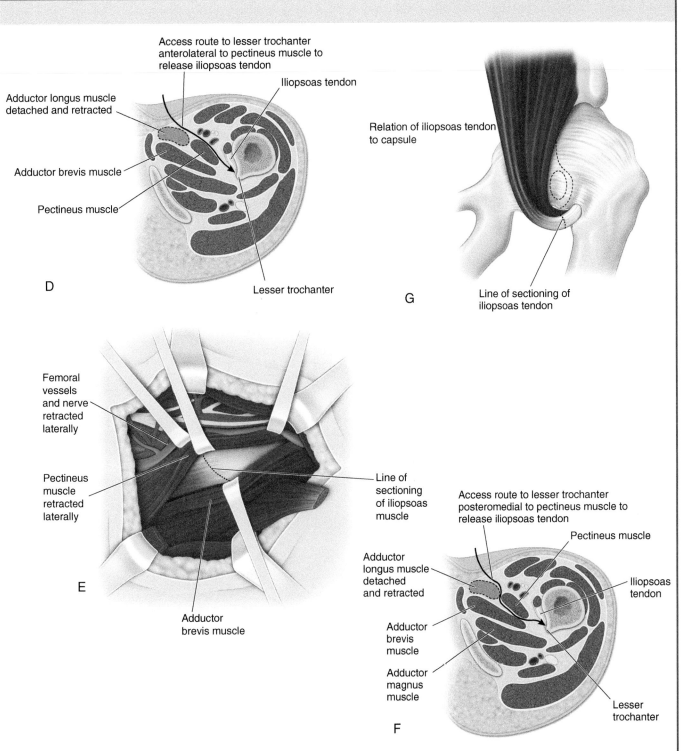

D, Transverse section showing the approach to the hip anterior to the pectineus.

Approach Medial to the Pectineus

E and **F,** The hip can also be approached by a route that is posteromedial to the pectineus muscle. The pectineus muscle is retracted laterally to protect the femoral vessels and nerve, and the adductor brevis muscle is retracted medially, thereby bringing the iliopsoas tendon into view at its insertion to the lesser trochanter. A Kelly clamp is passed under the iliopsoas tendon and opened slightly, and the tendon is sectioned.

G, With all of the medial approaches, the psoas tendon is sectioned and allowed to retract proximally, and the iliacus muscle fibers are gently elevated from the anterior aspect of the hip joint capsule.

Continued on following page

Procedure 2   **Medial Approach for Open Reduction of the Developmentally Dislocated Hip, cont'd**

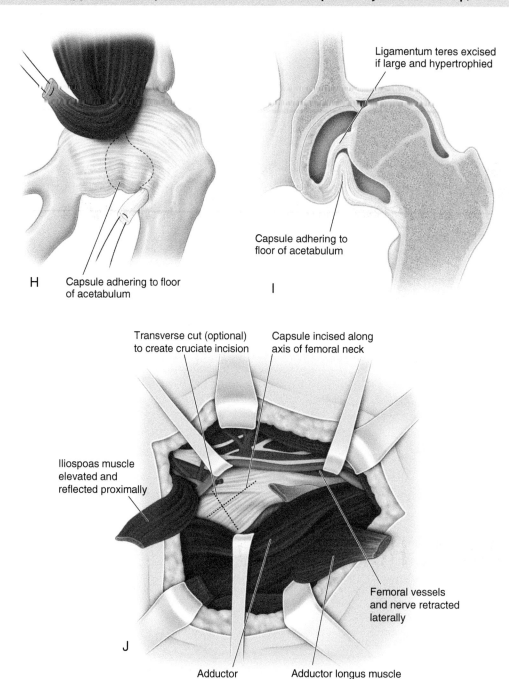

H   Capsule adhering to floor
           of acetabulum

Ligamentum teres excised
if large and hypertrophied

Capsule adhering to
floor of acetabulum

I

Transverse cut (optional)   Capsule incised along
to create cruciate incision   axis of femoral neck

Iliospoas muscle
elevated and
reflected proximally

Femoral vessels
and nerve retracted
laterally

J

Adductor   Adductor longus muscle
magnus muscle   detached and retracted

H and **I,** The inferior part of the capsule and the transverse ligament are pulled upward with the femoral head. The capsule may adhere to the floor of the acetabulum, and the ligamentum teres is enlarged and usually needs to be removed to better visualize and reduce the femoral head.

J, The capsule is opened with an incision that is parallel to the acetabular margin. It is best to make a small stab in the capsule, insert a small hemostat, and then complete the incision using the hemostat to protect the femoral head. In the drawing, a cruciate cut is shown; however, a single incision parallel to the acetabular margin is usually sufficient.

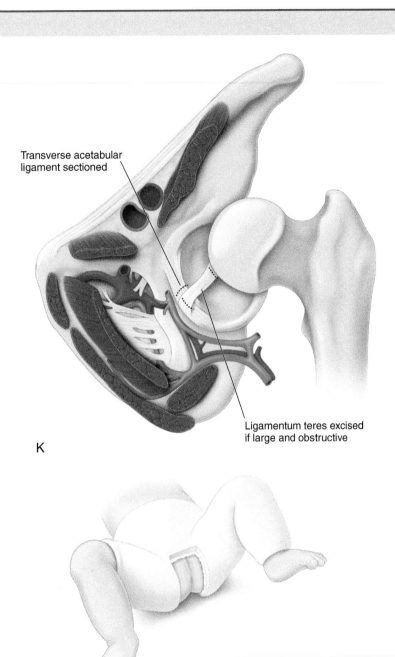

Transverse acetabular
ligament sectioned

Ligamentum teres excised
if large and obstructive

K

L

K, The transverse acetabular ligament is sectioned, and the ligamentum teres is excised. The hypertrophied pulvinar is also removed.

After this step, the femoral head should be easily reduced underneath the limbus. If the head does not reduce easily, the medial capsule and the transverse acetabular ligament should be released more thoroughly. Reduction can be maintained by holding the hip in 30 degrees of abduction, 90 to 100 degrees of flexion, and neutral rotation. It is not necessary to repair the capsule. The wound is closed in the usual fashion.

L, A one-and-one-half-hip spica cast is applied with the hip in 100 degrees of flexion, 30 degrees of abduction, and neutral rotation. During the application and setting of the cast, medially directed pressure is applied over the greater trochanter with the palm. The surgeon should be certain that the hip is not placed in maximal abduction to avoid excess pressure on the femoral head.

Postoperative Care

The cast is changed at 6-week intervals, with a total duration of cast immobilization of approximately 3 months.

Procedure 3   **Open Reduction of Developmental Hip Dislocation Through the Anterolateral Approach**

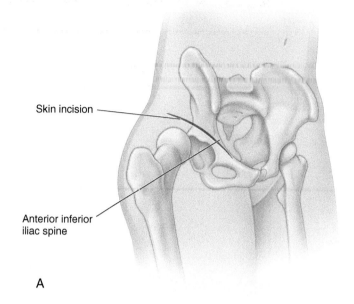

Skin incision

Anterior inferior
iliac spine

A

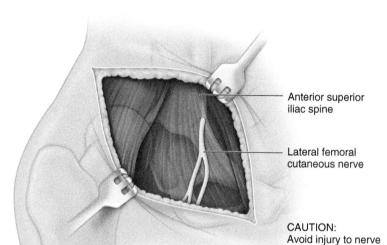

Anterior superior
iliac spine

Lateral femoral
cutaneous nerve

CAUTION:
Avoid injury to nerve

B

Operative Technique

A, The patient is placed supine with a roll under the hip. The entire lower limb and the affected half of the pelvis are prepared and draped to allow for the free motion of the hip.

The skin incision is an oblique "bikini" incision. The incision formerly used over the iliac crest produces an unsightly scar, whereas the bikini incision affords excellent exposure and cosmesis. The anterior inferior iliac spine is palpated and marked. The incision begins approximately two thirds of the distance from the greater trochanter to the iliac crest, crosses the inferior spine, and extends 1 or 2 cm beyond the inferior spine.

B, The incision is then retracted over the iliac crest, and the dissection is carried down to the apophysis of the crest.

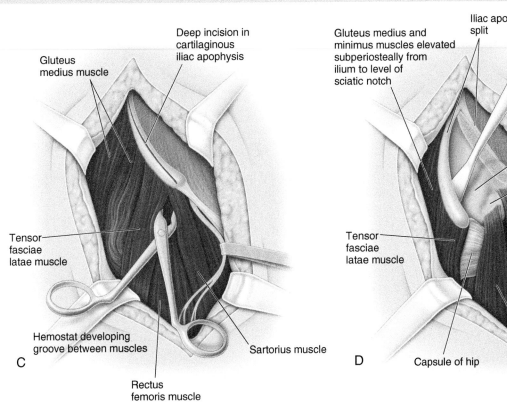

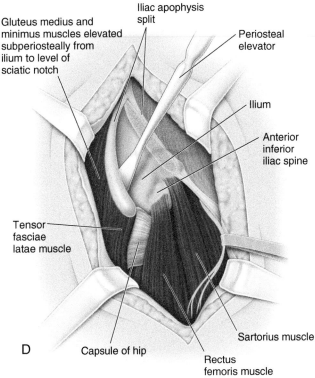

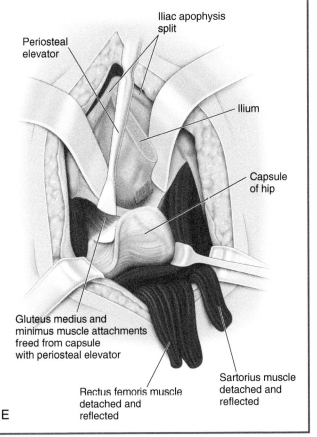

C, Anteriorly, the tensor–sartorius interval is bluntly dissected beginning distally and working proximally. The lateral femoral cutaneous nerve appears just medial to this interval and just distal to the inferior iliac spine, and it should be protected. The interval is widened with blunt dissection, and the rectus femoris is identified as it inserts on the anterior inferior iliac spine.

D, The iliac apophysis is now split with a scalpel or cautery down to the bone of the crest. With the help of periosteal elevators, the iliac crest is exposed subperiosteally. The surgeon must be careful to keep the periosteum intact because it protects the iliac muscles and prevents bleeding. Bleeding points on the iliac wings should be controlled with bone wax, even if the bleeding points appear to be small. A dry wound makes subsequent steps in the procedure easier. Further subperiosteal dissection clears the sartorius medially and the tensor laterally, thus exposing the rectus femoris as it arises from the anterior inferior spine.

E, The rectus femoris is elevated from the hip capsule, and the straight and reflected heads are identified, tagged, and sectioned. The hip capsule is exposed laterally, first with the aid of a periosteal elevator to clear muscle attachments from the capsule. Next, the medial portion of the capsule is exposed, again by using a periosteal elevator to dissect between the capsule and the iliopsoas tendon. Flexing the hip relaxes the iliopsoas and helps with the gaining of medial exposure. The capsule beneath the iliopsoas is exposed, and strong medial retraction with Army-Navy retractors is necessary to access the true acetabulum.

Continued on following page

Procedure 3 Open Reduction of Developmental Hip Dislocation Through the Anterolateral Approach, cont'd

F, If the iliopsoas tendon cannot be retracted, it may need to be sectioned.

G, When medial exposure is adequate, the capsule is opened with a knife. A hemostat is inserted into the capsule, and the capsule is opened over the instrument and parallel to the acetabular margin, leaving a 5-mm margin of capsule. This incision should extend medially all the way to the transverse acetabular ligament and laterally to above the greater trochanter. A second capsular incision is made down the femoral neck to form a T.

H, The capsule edges are grasped with Kocher clamps, and a blunt probe is inserted to visualize the acetabulum. The hip should be flexed and externally rotated to open up the acetabulum. The ligamentum teres is elevated with a right-angle clamp and followed to the depths of the acetabulum. This step is essential; many a surgeon has mistaken a false acetabulum for the true acetabulum.

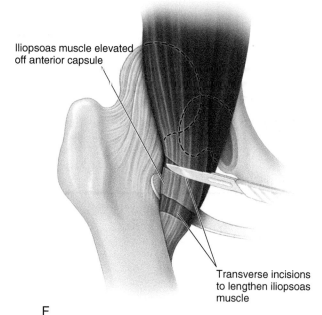

Iliopsoas muscle elevated off anterior capsule

Transverse incisions to lengthen iliopsoas muscle

F

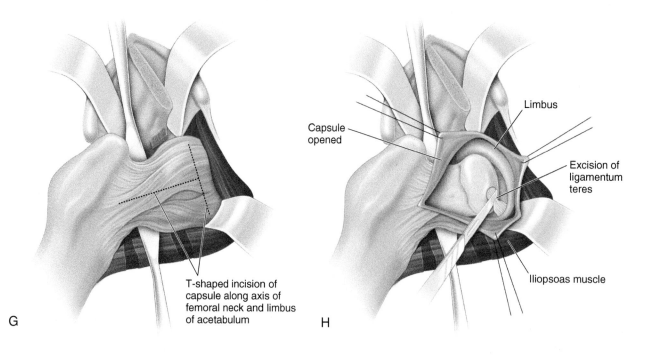

T-shaped incision of capsule along axis of femoral neck and limbus of acetabulum

G

Capsule opened

Limbus

Excision of ligamentum teres

Iliopsoas muscle

H

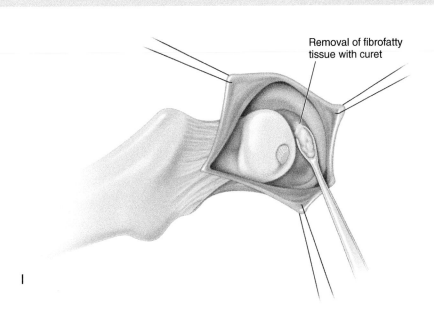

Removal of fibrofatty
tissue with curet

I

I, The ligamentum teres is cut free from its base in the acetabulum with scissors. The labrum of the acetabulum may initially appear to be folded into the acetabulum, especially when the head is reduced. This usually indicates that the medial obstacles to reduction (i.e., the capsule, the iliopsoas, and the transverse ligament) have been inadequately released. After more thorough release medially, the head should be reducible beneath the labrum, which will elevate the labrum out of the acetabulum. The excision of the labrum is almost never necessary.

Next, the surgeon inspects and determines (1) the depth of the acetabulum and the inclination of its roof; (2) the shape of the femoral head and the smoothness and condition of the articular hyaline cartilage covering it; (3) the degree of antetorsion of the femoral neck; and (4) the stability of the hip after reduction. The femoral head is placed in the acetabulum under direct vision by flexing, abducting, and medially rotating the hip while applying traction and gentle pressure against the greater trochanter. This maneuver is reversed to redislocate the hip. The position of the hip when the femoral head comes out of the acetabulum is determined and noted in the operative report. If necessary, sterile 4-0 or 5-0 suture wire is rolled into a circle and placed against the cartilaginous femoral head to delineate it, the hip is reduced, and radiographs are obtained; the wire is then removed. If the hip joint is unstable or if, after reduction under direct vision, the femoral head is insufficiently covered superiorly and anteriorly, the surgeon should decide whether to perform a Salter innominate osteotomy or a derotation osteotomy of the proximal femur at this time.

Continued on following page

Procedure 3 Open Reduction of Developmental Hip Dislocation Through the Anterolateral Approach, cont'd

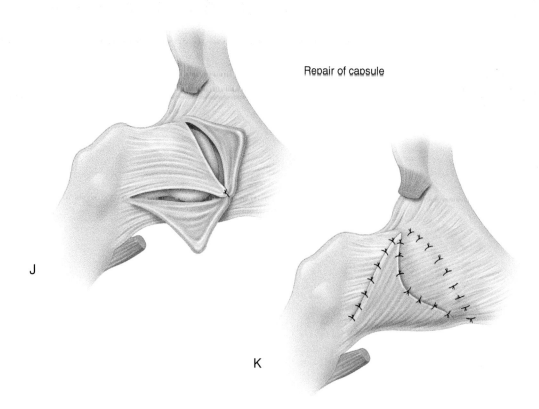

Repair of capsule

J

K

J and **K,** A careful capsuloplasty is performed next. It is very important to keep the femoral head in its anatomic position in the acetabulum. With the femoral head reduced, the hip joint is held by a second assistant in 30 degrees of abduction, 30 to 45 degrees of flexion, and 20 to 30 degrees of medial rotation throughout the remainder of the operation. The degree of medial rotation depends on the severity of antetorsion.

The large, redundant, superior pocket of the capsule should be obliterated via the plication and overlapping of its free edges. The capsule should also be tightened medially and anteriorly with a vest-over-pants closure. If this closure is too lax and redundant, a portion may be excised. With the hip dislocated, nonabsorbable sutures are passed through the medial portion of the capsule, which is still attached above the acetabulum. The needles are left on the sutures and held with clamps. The hip is reduced, and the superolateral segment of the capsule is brought medially and distally with a Kocher clamp; this holds the hip internally rotated and deeply seated in the acetabulum. The sutures are passed through the capsule in this position and tied. Any redundant capsule is imbricated over this closure with nonabsorbable sutures. The two halves of the iliac apophysis are sutured together over the iliac crest. The rectus femoris and sartorius muscles are resutured to

their origins. The wound is then closed in routine manner. An anteroposterior radiograph of the hips is obtained to ensure a concentric reduction before a one-and-one-half-hip spica cast is applied. The roll beneath the patient's hip should be removed when the radiograph is made to obtain a true anteroposterior view of the pelvis. The cast is applied with the hip in approximately 45 degrees of abduction, 60 to 70 degrees of flexion, and 20 to 30 degrees of medial rotation. The knee is always flexed at 45 to 60 degrees to relax the hamstrings and to control rotation in the cast.

Postoperative Care

The patient is immobilized in a one-and-one-half-hip spica cast for 6 weeks. After 6 weeks, the patient is examined under anesthesia, and a Petrie type of cast is applied. This consists of long-leg plasters that are connected by one or two bars, with the hips abducted 45 degrees and internally rotated 15 degrees. The cast allows for the flexion and extension of the hips while the reduction is maintained by the abduction and internal rotation. The cast is removed in the clinic after 4 weeks. Weight bearing is allowed while the child is in the cast. If stability is uncertain, a second spica cast may be appropriate.

Procedure 4   Femoral Shortening and Derotation Osteotomy Combined With Open Reduction of the Hip
(see Video 2 and Video 3)

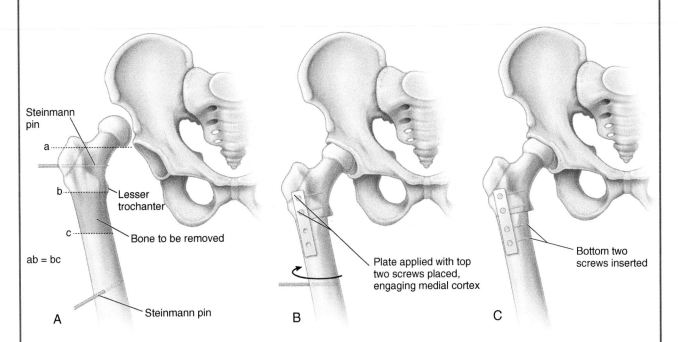

A femoral shortening and derotation osteotomy procedure is performed through a separate lateral longitudinal incision, although other surgeons may use different approaches. The exposure of the upper femoral shaft through a separate longitudinal incision of the upper thigh is technically simpler; there is less bleeding, and the scars are aesthetically more attractive. It is vital to expose a sufficient length of the upper femoral shaft subperiosteally.

With an irreducible dislocation, femoral shortening facilitates reduction; when reduction is difficult because of increasing pressure on the femoral head, it also decompresses the hip.

Operative Technique

A, Femoral shortening is necessary to reduce pressure on the reduced femoral head, which is known to cause avascular necrosis of the hip. The amount of shortening may be estimated from the preoperative supine radiograph by measuring the distance from the bottom of the femoral head to the floor of the acetabulum (*a* to *b*). The distance from *b* to *c* must equal the distance from *a* to *b*. With higher dislocations, however, this may overestimate the needed shortening. The dissection for the open reduction, including clearing the acetabulum, is performed before the transection of the femur. A trial reduction gives the surgeon a feel for the tightness of the muscles and other foreshortened structures, thus allowing for another estimate of the amount of shortening needed.

A longitudinal mark is made with the saw along the anterior aspect of the femoral shaft. This serves as an orientation mark for femoral rotation. Steinmann pins may also be placed transversely through the femur above and below the proposed osteotomy.

B, The femur is transected just below the lesser trochanter. The hip is reduced, and the distal femoral shaft is aligned with the proximal shaft. The amount of overlap is noted, which gives the surgeon the final estimate of shortening necessary; this is usually between 1 and 2 cm. This overlap is marked on the distal fragment, and the femoral shaft is transected again at that level. A four-hole plate is attached to the proximal fragment, and the distal shaft is held to the plate with a Verbrugge clamp.

C, The reduction is completed and assessed with regard to femoral rotation and adequacy of shortening. As a rule, the degree of hip decompression is adequate if the surgeon can, with a moderate force, distract the reduced femoral head 3 or 4 mm from the acetabulum. With the rotation marks aligned, the position of the lower extremity should be in moderate internal rotation. Derotation is done only when the internal rotation position is severe. The remaining screws are placed to fix the plate to the distal fragment.

The lateral thigh wound is closed in the usual manner. The repair of the hip capsule as well as other steps are illustrated in Procedure 3 on page 8.

Postoperative Care

Postoperative care is similar to that which occurs after open reduction of the hip. The plate can be removed after 6 months, when the osteotomy has solidly healed.

Procedure 5   **Intertrochanteric Varus Osteotomy and Internal Fixation With a Blade Plate**

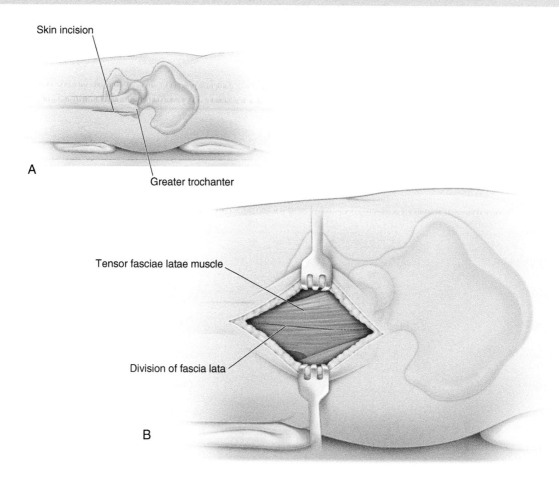

Skin incision

Greater trochanter

A

Tensor fasciae latae muscle

Division of fascia lata

B

Operative Technique

A, The operation is performed with the child supine on a radiolucent operating table. It is imperative to have image-intensifier radiographic control. Some surgeons prefer to operate on an older child on a fracture table because it is technically easier to obtain a lateral radiograph of the hip. A straight, midlateral, longitudinal incision is made beginning at the tip of the greater trochanter and extending distally parallel to the femur for a distance of 10 to 12 cm. The subcutaneous tissue is divided in line with the skin incision.

B, The fascia lata is exposed by deepening the dissection. It is first divided with a scalpel, and it is then split longitudinally with scissors in the direction of its fibers. The fascia lata should be divided posterior to the tensor fasciae latae to avoid splitting the muscle.

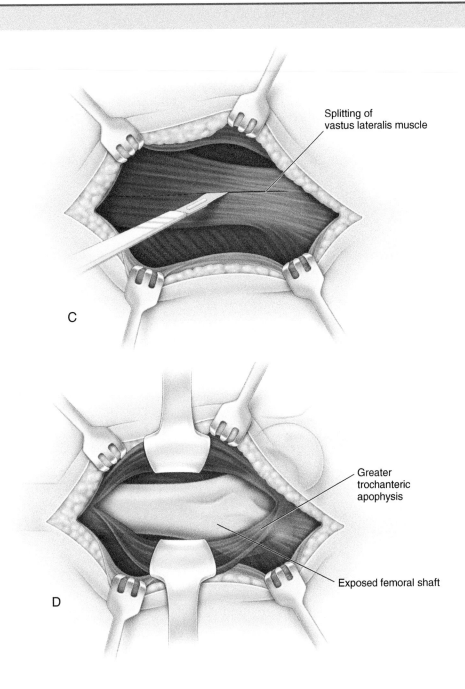

Splitting of
vastus lateralis muscle

C

Greater
trochanteric
apophysis

Exposed femoral shaft

D

C, With retraction, the vastus lateralis muscle is visualized. Next, the anterolateral region of the proximal femur and the trochanteric area are exposed. It is vital to not injure the greater trochanteric growth plate. The origin of the vastus lateralis muscle is divided transversely from the inferior border of the greater trochanter down to the posterolateral surface of the femur. The vastus lateralis muscle fibers are elevated from the lateral intramuscular septum and the tendinous insertion of the gluteus maximus. **D,** The lateral femoral surface is exposed by subperiosteal dissection. The greater trochanteric apophysis should not be disturbed.

Continued on following page

Procedure 5   Intertrochanteric Varus Osteotomy and Internal Fixation With a Blade Plate, cont'd

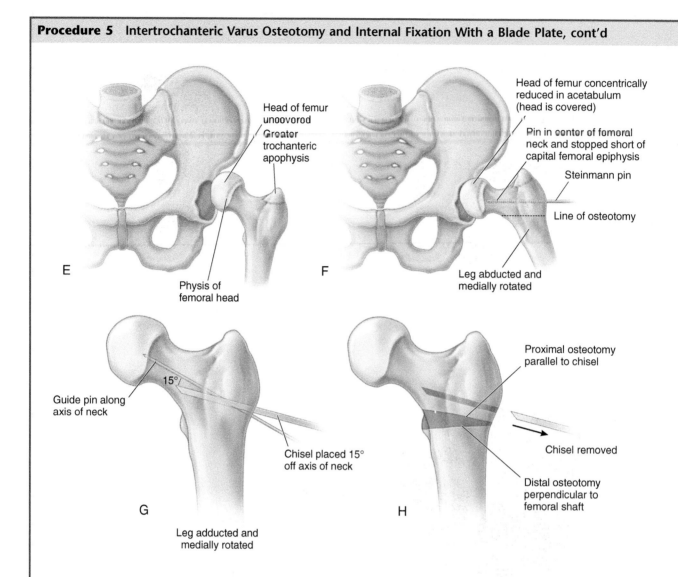

E, Head of femur uncovered
Greater trochanteric apophysis
Physis of femoral head

F, Head of femur concentrically reduced in acetabulum (head is covered)
Pin in center of femoral neck and stopped short of capital femoral epiphysis
Steinmann pin
Line of osteotomy
Leg abducted and medially rotated

G, Guide pin along axis of neck
15°
Chisel placed 15° off axis of neck
Leg adducted and medially rotated

H, Proximal osteotomy parallel to chisel
Chisel removed
Distal osteotomy perpendicular to femoral shaft

E and F, The femoral head is centered concentrically in the acetabulum by abducting and medially rotating the hip, and its position is checked with an image intensifier. Immediately distal to the apophyseal growth plate of the greater trochanter, a 3-mm Steinmann pin is inserted through the lateral cortex of the femoral shaft parallel to the floor of the operating room and at a right angle to the median plane of the patient. The pin is drilled medially along the longitudinal axis of the femoral neck and stops short of the capital femoral physis. This position of the proximal femur can be reproduced at any time during the operation by placing the Steinmann pin horizontally parallel to the floor and at 90 degrees to the longitudinal axis of the patient. This is a very dependable and simple method for properly orienting the proximal femur.

G, The chisel for the blade plate is placed at an angle that is determined as follows: if the chisel paralleled the guide pin, the 90-degree blade plate would produce a 90-degree neck–shaft angle. In this case, we sought to produce a neck–shaft angle of 105 degrees. Thus a chisel placed 15 degrees off of the guide pin's axis adds 15 degrees to a 90-degree neck–shaft angle, thereby resulting in a 105-degree final angle.

H, The osteotomy cuts are made while the chisel is in place. The proximal osteotomy is parallel to the chisel, and the distal osteotomy is perpendicular to the femoral shaft.

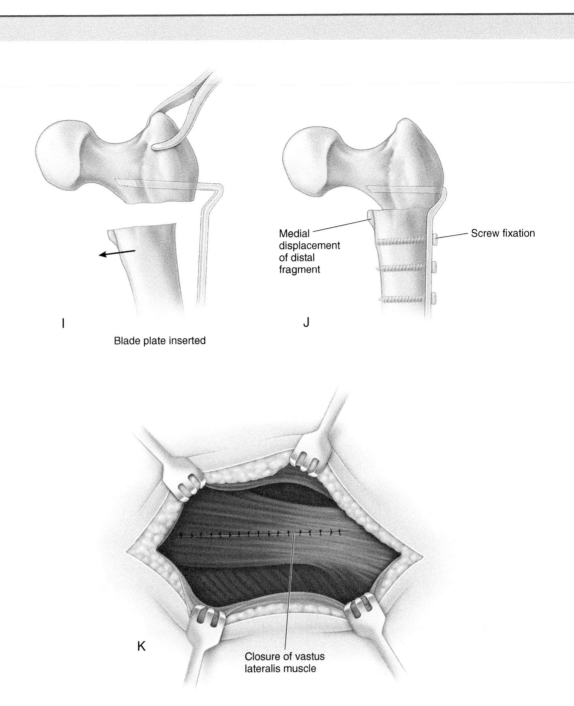

Blade plate inserted

Medial displacement of distal fragment — Screw fixation

I

J

K — Closure of vastus lateralis muscle

I, After the osteotomized triangle is removed, the chisel is removed, and the blade plate is inserted. Careful control of the proximal fragment and clear visualization of the entry site of the chisel facilitate the placement of the blade.

J, The blade plate is fully seated and secured with screws that are drilled and tapped. The angulation of the plate produces medial displacement of the femoral shaft, which is extremely important to the biomechanics of the hip. Failure to displace the distal fragments medially results in the lateral prominence of the plate and the widening of the groin.

K, The vastus lateralis and fascia lata are closed with running sutures. Subcutaneous and skin closure with absorbable sutures completes the procedure.

Postoperative Care

The osteotomy is stable when the bone is of normal strength. In reliable patients, cast immobilization is not necessary. For less reliable children, those with osteopenic bone, and always when an open reduction has been performed, 6 weeks in a spica cast are required.

Procedure 6   Greater Trochanteric Epiphysiodesis

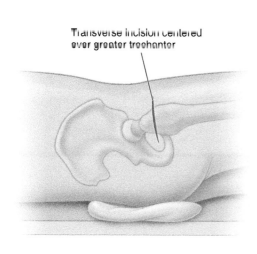

Transverse incision centered over greater trochanter

A

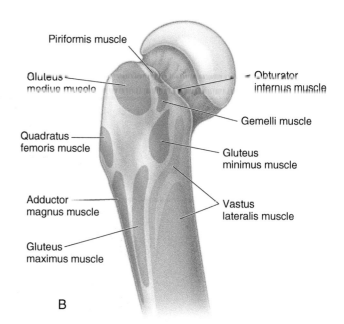

Piriformis muscle
Gluteus medius muscle
Obturator internus muscle
Gemelli muscle
Quadratus femoris muscle
Gluteus minimus muscle
Adductor magnus muscle
Vastus lateralis muscle
Gluteus maximus muscle

B

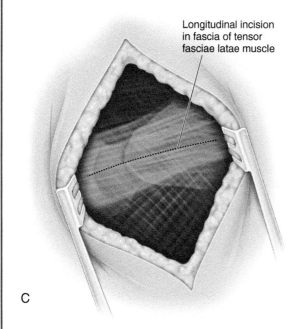

Longitudinal incision in fascia of tensor fasciae latae muscle

C

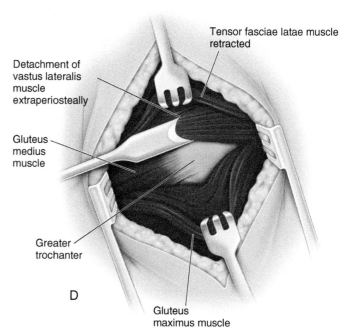

Tensor fasciae latae muscle retracted
Detachment of vastus lateralis muscle extraperiosteally
Gluteus medius muscle
Greater trochanter
Gluteus maximus muscle

D

Operative Technique

A, The child is placed supine with a sandbag under the ipsilateral hip. The entire lower limb, hip, and pelvis are prepared and draped to permit the free passive motion of the hip. A transverse incision that is 5 to 7 cm long is centered over the epiphysis of the greater trochanter. If desired, a longitudinal incision may be made, especially if the distal transfer of the greater trochanter is anticipated in the future.

B, The site of origin of the vastus lateralis from the upper part of the intertrochanteric line, the anteroinferior border of the greater trochanter, the lateral tip of the gluteal tuberosity, and the upper part of the lateral tip of the linea aspera are shown.

C, The subcutaneous tissue is divided in line with the skin incision, and the wound edges are retracted. A longitudinal incision is made in the fascia of the tensor fasciae latae muscle.

D, The tensor fasciae latae muscle is retracted anteriorly, and the origin of the vastus lateralis is detached and elevated extraperiosteally.

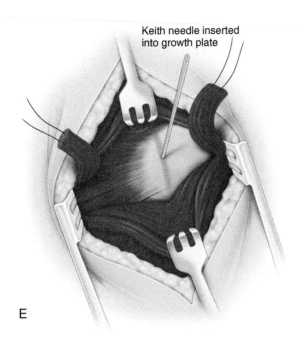

Keith needle inserted
into growth plate

E

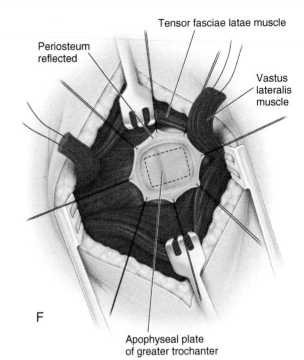

Tensor fasciae latae muscle

Periosteum
reflected

Vastus
lateralis
muscle

Apophyseal plate
of greater trochanter

F

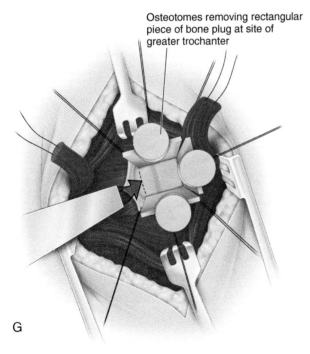

Osteotomes removing rectangular
piece of bone plug at site of
greater trochanter

G

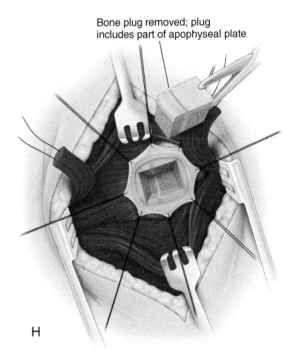

Bone plug removed; plug
includes part of apophyseal plate

H

E, A Keith needle is inserted into the soft growth plate of the greater trochanteric epiphysis. Anteroposterior radiographs are obtained to verify the position of the Keith needle and the growth plate. (Many surgeons will perform the arrest by removing the physeal cartilage with a curet that is controlled with radiographic image intensification.)

F, The periosteum is divided by one longitudinal and two horizontal incisions. The *dotted rectangle* marks the bone plug to be removed and turned around. This rectangle is 2 cm long and 1.25 cm wide. In a smaller child, the rectangle is 1 cm (⅖ inch) long and 0.6 cm (⅕ inch) wide. **G** and **H,** With straight osteotomies, the bone plug is removed. Note that the growth plate is in the proximal third of the rectangle.

Continued on following page

Procedure 6 Greater Trochanteric Epiphysiodesis, cont'd

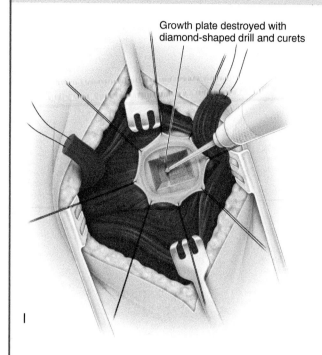

Growth plate destroyed with diamond-shaped drill and curets

I

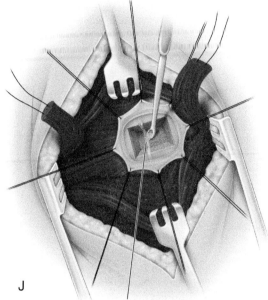

J

Cancellous bone (from proximal femoral shaft) placed in cleared growth plate defect

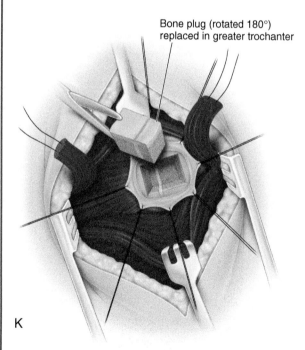

Bone plug (rotated 180°) replaced in greater trochanter

K

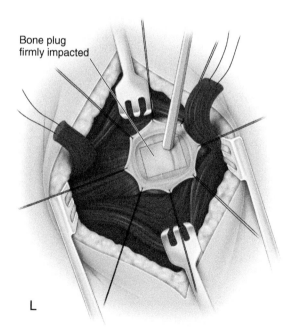

Bone plug firmly impacted

L

I, A diamond-shaped drill and curets are used to destroy the growth plate. The operator should be careful to not enter the trochanteric fossa and injure the circulation to the femoral head.

J, With a curved osteotome, cancellous bone is removed from the proximal femoral shaft and packed into the defect at the site of the growth plate.

K and **L,** The bone plug is rotated 180 degrees, replaced in the defect in the greater trochanter, and, with an impactor and mallet, securely seated.

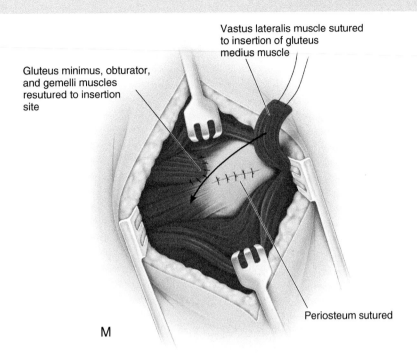

Gluteus minimus, obturator, and gemelli muscles resutured to insertion site

Vastus lateralis muscle sutured to insertion of gluteus medius muscle

Periosteum sutured

M

M, The muscles are resutured to their insertion sites, and the vastus lateralis is attached to the gluteus medius and minimus tendons at their insertion sites after the closure of the periosteum. The fascia lata is closed with interrupted sutures, and the wound is closed with interrupted and subcuticular sutures. It is not necessary to immobilize the hip in a cast.

Postoperative Care

The patient is allowed out of bed on the first postoperative day as soon as he or she is comfortable. The patient is discharged to home within a few days and instructed to protect the limb that was operated on by using a three-point crutch gait for 3 to 4 weeks.

Procedure 7   Distal and Lateral Transfer of the Greater Trochanter

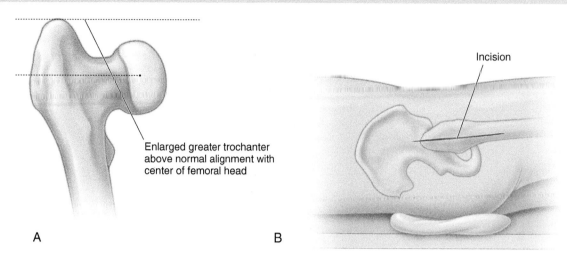

Enlarged greater trochanter
above normal alignment with
center of femoral head

A

Incision

B

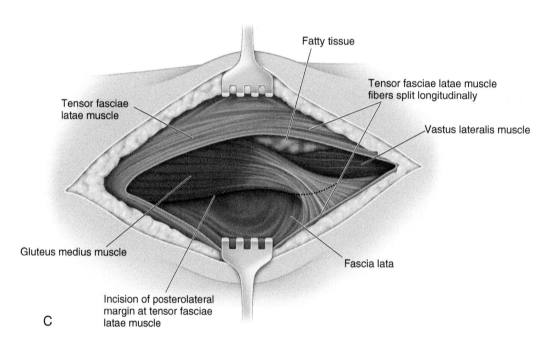

Fatty tissue

Tensor fasciae latae muscle
fibers split longitudinally

Tensor fasciae
latae muscle

Vastus lateralis muscle

Gluteus medius muscle

Fascia lata

Incision of posterolateral
margin at tensor fasciae
latae muscle

C

Operative Technique

A and **B,** The patient is placed on the fracture table with the affected hip in a neutral position with regard to adduction and abduction and in 20 to 30 degrees of medial rotation to bring the greater trochanter forward to facilitate exposure. The opposite hip is placed in 40 degrees of abduction. Image-intensifier anteroposterior fluoroscopy is used to show the femoral head and neck, the greater trochanter, and the upper femoral shaft. The hip should be rotated medially so that the greater trochanter is seen in profile and not superimposed on the femoral neck. It is crucial to see the trochanteric fossa. The affected hip and the upper two thirds of the thigh are prepared and draped in the usual manner.

A straight, lateral, longitudinal incision is made from the tip of the greater trochanter and extended distally for 10 cm. The subcutaneous tissue is divided in line with the skin incision.

C, The fascia lata is split longitudinally in the direction of its fibers.

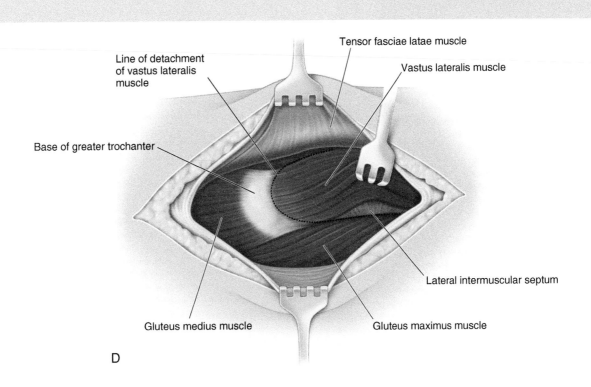

D

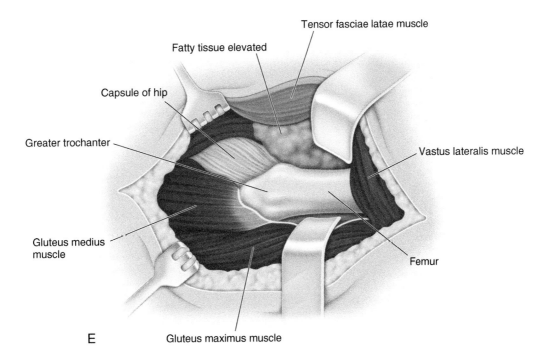

E

D and **E,** The vastus lateralis is detached proximally from the abductor tubercle by a proximally based horseshoe-shaped incision and elevated subperiosteally from the femoral shaft for 5 to 7 cm. The vastus lateralis should be elevated over its entire width.

Continued on following page

Procedure 7   Distal and Lateral Transfer of the Greater Trochanter, cont'd

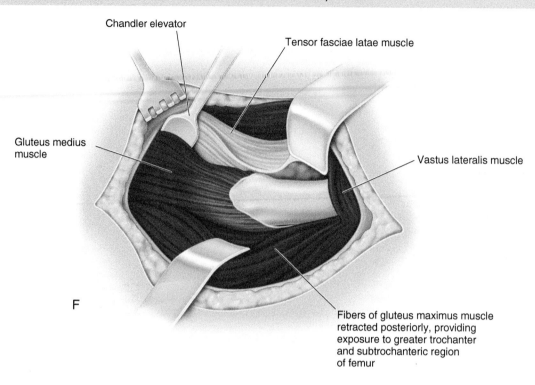

Chandler elevator

Tensor fasciae latae muscle

Gluteus medius muscle

Vastus lateralis muscle

Fibers of gluteus maximus muscle retracted posteriorly, providing exposure to greater trochanter and subtrochanteric region of femur

F

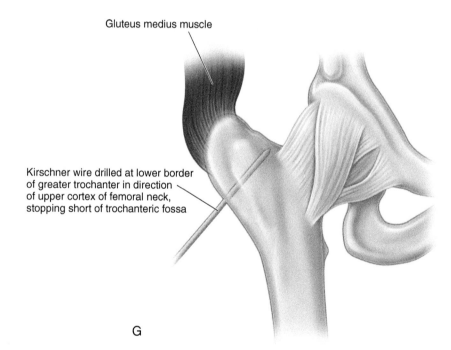

Gluteus medius muscle

Kirschner wire drilled at lower border of greater trochanter in direction of upper cortex of femoral neck, stopping short of trochanteric fossa

G

F, The anterior border of the gluteus medius is identified, and a blunt elevator retractor is introduced beneath its deep surface; it is pointed in the direction of the trochanteric fossa.

G, At this time, to orient the plane of the trochanteric osteotomy properly, a smooth Kirschner wire is inserted at the level of the abductor tubercle; it points to the trochanteric fossa along a line that is continuous with the upper cortex of the femoral neck. Radiography with image intensification verifies the proper level and depth of the guide wire. The point of the Kirschner wire must not protrude through the medial cortex into the trochanteric fossa.

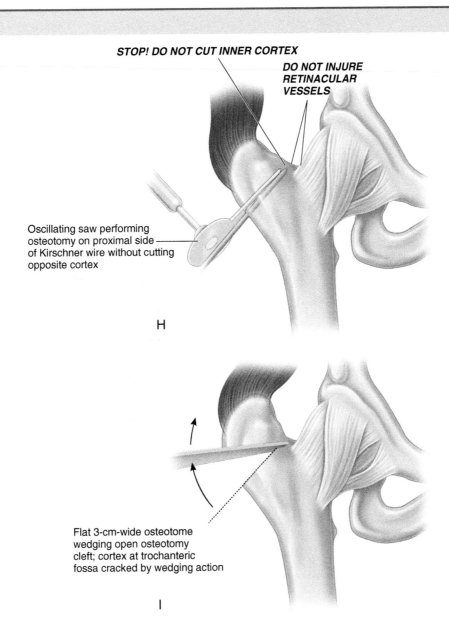

STOP! DO NOT CUT INNER CORTEX

DO NOT INJURE RETINACULAR VESSELS

Oscillating saw performing osteotomy on proximal side of Kirschner wire without cutting opposite cortex

H

Flat 3-cm-wide osteotome wedging open osteotomy cleft; cortex at trochanteric fossa cracked by wedging action

I

H, A blunt, flat retractor is placed beneath the posterior border of the greater trochanter to protect the soft tissues. The previously applied anterior retractor protects the soft tissues ventrally. With a 2- to 3-cm-wide reciprocating saw, the greater trochanter is divided in the anteroposterior direction, following the proximal border of the Kirschner wire. The cut is stopped 3 mm short of the medial cortex of the trochanteric fossa. Injury to the vessels in the trochanteric fossa must be avoided to prevent necrosis of the femoral head.

I, Next, a 3-mm-wide flat osteotome is driven through the osteotomy cleft, and the osteotomy site is wedged open by moving the handle of the osteotome craniad. By applying leverage with the osteotome in the cleft, the operator produces a greenstick fracture of the medial cortex.

Continued on following page

Procedure 7   Distal and Lateral Transfer of the Greater Trochanter, cont'd

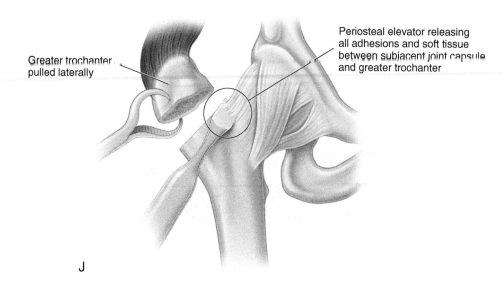

Greater trochanter pulled laterally

Periosteal elevator releasing all adhesions and soft tissue between subjacent joint capsule and greater trochanter

J

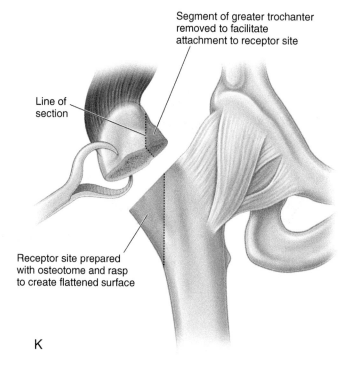

Segment of greater trochanter removed to facilitate attachment to receptor site

Line of section

Receptor site prepared with osteotome and rasp to create flattened surface

K

J, A large periosteal elevator is placed deep into the osteotomy cleft; this cleft is opened up medially by gently levering the handle up and down. The trochanteric fragment is lifted superolaterally with a Lewin bone clamp, and adhesions between the joint capsule and the medial aspect of the greater trochanter are released. This must be done very carefully to avoid injuring retinacular blood vessels in the capsule. Do not fracture the greater trochanter. Mobilization is sufficient when, with lateral and distal traction placed on the greater trochanter, the muscle response is elastic; if there is still muscle resistance, it means that further adhesions are present that must be freed.

K, After sufficient mobilization of the greater trochanter, the recipient site on the lateral surface of the upper femoral shaft is prepared with a curved osteotome to create a flattened surface. The surgeon should not remove too much bone laterally. Next, the greater trochanter is displaced distally and laterally; with excessive femoral antetorsion, it may be moved slightly forward. If additional distal advancement is desired, the hip may be abducted on the fracture table.

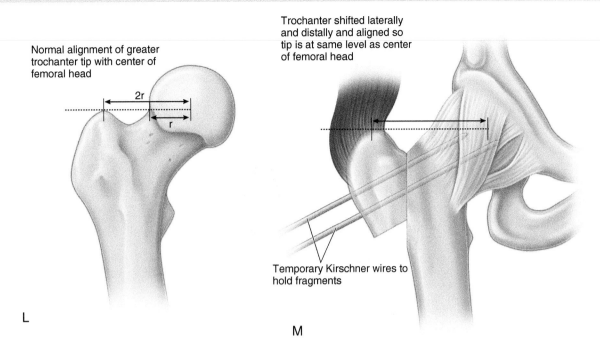

Normal alignment of greater trochanter tip with center of femoral head

2r

r

Trochanter shifted laterally and distally and aligned so tip is at same level as center of femoral head

Temporary Kirschner wires to hold fragments

L

M

L and M, The trochanter is held in the desired position and temporarily fixed to the femur with two threaded Kirschner wires of adequate size that are drilled upward and medially. At this point, the accuracy of the position of the greater trochanter is verified with image-intensifier radiography. As stated previously, the tip of the greater trochanter should be level with the center of the femoral head and at a distance from it of two to two-and-one-half times the radius of the femoral head. If there are problems with proper visualization, a long Kirschner wire is placed horizontally and parallel to both anterior superior iliac spines so that it crosses the center of the femoral head; the position of the tip of the greater trochanter is then checked.

N, Before osteosynthesis, the gluteal muscle is split in the direction of the fibers to expose the bone and to avoid muscle necrosis. The greater trochanter is fixed to the lateral surface of the upper femur with two lag screws (each equipped with a washer), which are directed medially and distally at 45-degree angles to counteract the pull of the hip abductors. For large trochanters, 6.5-mm cancellous screws with drill bits of appropriate size are used; with smaller trochanters, 3.2-mm screws are used. The outer cortex of the greater trochanter may be overdrilled. The tapping of the outer cortex is optional. The washers increase the surface area, help the operator to avoid cutting through the cortex, ensure more secure fixation, and allow for early motion. After both screws are inserted, the initial Kirschner wires are removed.

O, Alternatively, fixation can be achieved with two heavy, threaded Kirschner wires directed medially and upward. The resultant pull of the hip abductors through the direction of the wires provides a force that will compress the greater trochanter against the lateral surface of the femur. We do not recommend internal fixation with the use of this

method because screw fixation is more stable. However, in an obese or uncooperative patient, threaded Kirschner wires may be used in addition to screw fixation. Alternatively, a tension wire band may be used as described in Procedure 8 on page 29, "Lateral Advancement of the Greater Trochanter."

P, Final intraoperative radiographs are obtained to ensure that the trochanter has been advanced to the desired site. Next, the detached origin of the vastus lateralis is firmly sutured to the tendinous insertion of the gluteus medius and minimus muscles. This tension-band suture absorbs the pull of the hip abductors and reinforces the internal fixation of the greater trochanter. A suction drain is inserted, and the remainder of the wound is closed in routine fashion. The skin closure is subcuticular.

Postoperative Care

The patient is placed in split Russell traction or on an abduction pillow with each hip in 35 to 40 degrees of abduction. Active assisted exercises are begun as soon as the patient is comfortable. Adduction and excessive flexion of the hip should be avoided. Hip abduction exercises are performed with the patient in a supine position, which eliminates the effect of gravity. Sitting should be allowed gradually and with care because, with 60 to 90 degrees of hip flexion, the posterior fibers of the gluteus medius muscle exert a strong lateral rotary force on the greater trochanter and may loosen its fixation.

The patient is allowed out of bed on crutches when comfortable and should be instructed to walk using a three-point gait with partial weight bearing to protect the recently treated limb. The patient is discharged as soon as he or she is independent and secure on crutches. Three weeks after

Continued on following page

Procedure 7   **Distal and Lateral Transfer of the Greater Trochanter, cont'd**

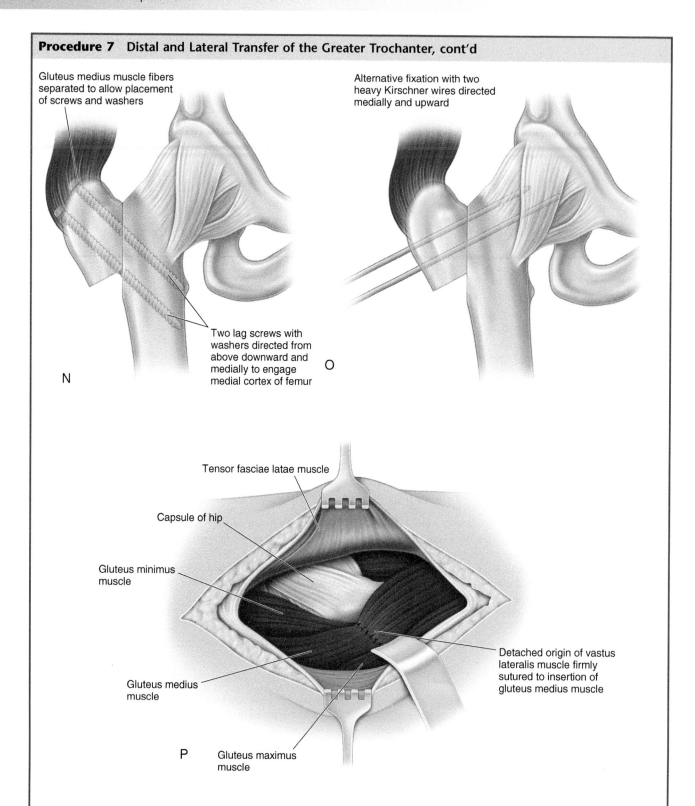

Gluteus medius muscle fibers separated to allow placement of screws and washers

Alternative fixation with two heavy Kirschner wires directed medially and upward

Two lag screws with washers directed from above downward and medially to engage medial cortex of femur

N

O

Tensor fasciae latae muscle

Capsule of hip

Gluteus minimus muscle

Gluteus medius muscle

Detached origin of vastus lateralis muscle firmly sutured to insertion of gluteus medius muscle

P   Gluteus maximus muscle

surgery, side-lying hip abduction exercises are started, and the child is allowed to sit and return to school. At 6 weeks, bony consolidation is usually adequate to begin the use of one crutch on the opposite side (to protect the operated hip) and to perform standing Trendelenburg exercises. One-crutch protection should be continued until the hip abductor muscles are normal or good with regard to motor strength and until the Trendelenburg sign is absent.

The screws are removed 3 to 6 months after surgery. During screw removal, the operator should be very careful to not damage the gluteus medius and minimus muscle fibers. After the removal of the screws, the hip is protected by three-point partial weight bearing on crutches for 2 to 3 weeks. Side-lying hip abduction exercises and standing Trendelenburg exercises are performed to regain the motor strength of the hip abductor muscles.

Procedure 8   Lateral Advancement of the Greater Trochanter

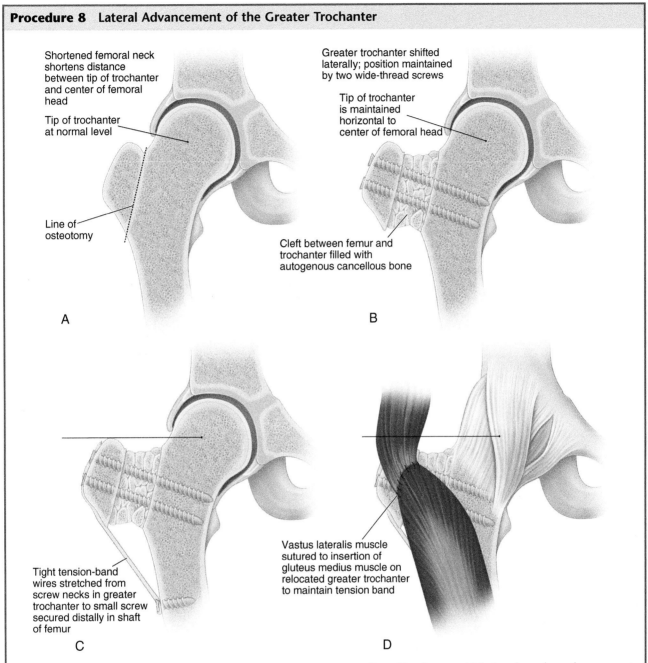

Shortened femoral neck shortens distance between tip of trochanter and center of femoral head

Tip of trochanter at normal level

Line of osteotomy

A

Greater trochanter shifted laterally; position maintained by two wide-thread screws

Tip of trochanter is maintained horizontal to center of femoral head

Cleft between femur and trochanter filled with autogenous cancellous bone

B

Tight tension-band wires stretched from screw necks in greater trochanter to small screw secured distally in shaft of femur

C

Vastus lateralis muscle sutured to insertion of gluteus medius muscle on relocated greater trochanter to maintain tension band

D

Operative Technique

A, The surgical exposure of the greater trochanter and the upper femoral shaft is similar to that for the distal and lateral transfer of the greater trochanter (see Procedure 7, **A** to **K,** on page 22).

B, The tip of the greater trochanter is at its normal level, so it is not necessary to advance it distally. It is kept horizontally level with the center of the femoral head, and its position is maintained by two wide-thread positional cancellous screws. The screws are inserted horizontally and perpendicular to the osteotomized lateral surface of the upper femur. The threads of these "positioning" screws grip the trochanter as well as the intertrochanteric region of the femur without compression. The cleft between the greater trochanter and the femur is filled with autogenous cancellous iliac bone, which is taken through a separate incision over the iliac apophysis.

C, Internal fixation is augmented by a taut tension band of heavy wire suture that extends from the neck of each trochanteric screw to a small unicortical screw that is anchored 6 cm distally in the femur. This wire tension band counteracts the pull of the hip abductors.

D, The detached vastus lateralis is then sutured to the insertion of the gluteus medius. The subcutaneous tissue and the skin are closed in the usual manner.

Postoperative Care

Postoperative care is similar to that used after the distal and lateral transfer of the greater trochanter (see Procedure 7 on page 22)

Procedure 9   Lateral Closing Wedge Valgization Osteotomy of the Proximal Femur With Distal and Lateral Advancement of the Greater Trochanter

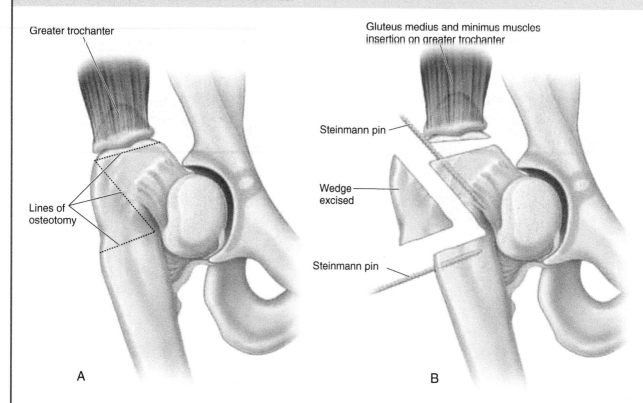

A

B

The greater trochanter and the upper femoral shaft are exposed with the use of the technique described in Procedure 7, steps **A** to **K,** on page 22. If the hip adductors are taut, they are released through a separate medial incision.

Operative Technique

A and **B,** First, the greater trochanter is osteotomized with the use of the technique described for distal and lateral advancement. Next, two threaded Steinmann pins are inserted to serve as guides for the level and angle of the osteotomy. The apex of the osteotomy stops 1 cm short of the medial cortex. The length of the base of the wedge depends on the degree of correction of the coxa vara that is required. The wedge of bone is resected with an oscillating saw.
C, With a straight osteotome and leverage from the pins anchored in the femur, a greenstick fracture is produced in the medial cortex, thereby converting the osteotomy to a short-stemmed Y.

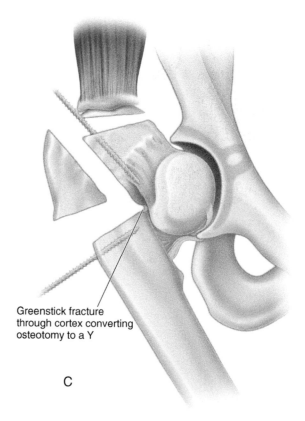

C

D, The osteotomy gap is closed by bringing the two Steinmann pins together and by aligning the neck, shaft, and the greater trochanter at a preoperatively determined angle.

E, The greater trochanter is transfixed with a threaded Steinmann pin that is driven into the neck of the femur.

F, The three fragments are then fixed with a prebent trochanteric hook plate and screws.

Postoperative Care

Care after this operation is similar to that provided after the Wagner intertrochanteric double osteotomy.

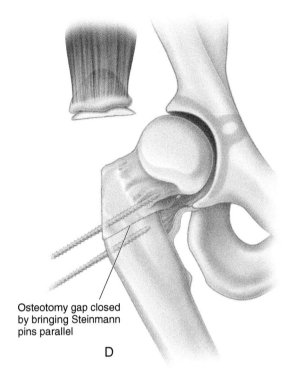

Osteotomy gap closed by bringing Steinmann pins parallel

D

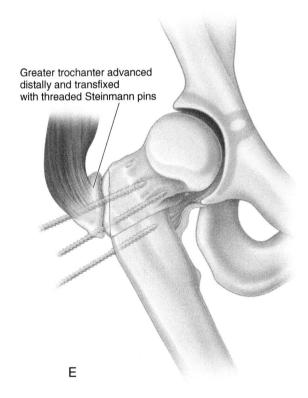

Greater trochanter advanced distally and transfixed with threaded Steinmann pins

E

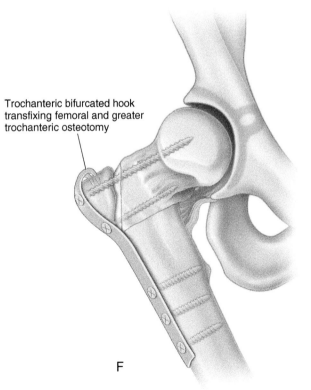

Trochanteric bifurcated hook transfixing femoral and greater trochanteric osteotomy

F

Procedure 10 **Pemberton Osteotomy** (see Video 4)

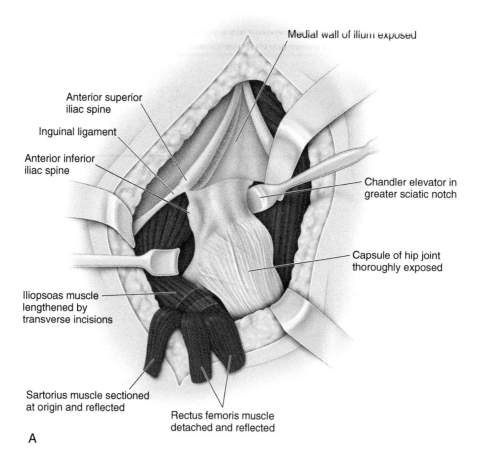

Medial wall of ilium exposed

Anterior superior
iliac spine

Inguinal ligament

Anterior inferior
iliac spine

Chandler elevator in
greater sciatic notch

Capsule of hip joint
thoroughly exposed

Iliopsoas muscle
lengthened by
transverse incisions

Sartorius muscle sectioned
at origin and reflected

Rectus femoris muscle
detached and reflected

A

The skin of the affected side of the abdomen and pelvis and the entire lower limb are prepared with the patient lying on his or her side, and the patient is draped to allow for free hip motion during surgery. Next, the patient is placed completely supine. The operation is performed on a radiolucent operating table. It is imperative to have image-intensification fluoroscopic and radiographic control.

Operative Technique

A, The medial and lateral walls of the ilium and the hip joint are exposed through an anterolateral iliofemoral approach. The cartilaginous apophysis of the ilium is split in accordance with the Salter technique. The sartorius muscle is sectioned at its origin from the anterior superior iliac spine, tagged with 2-0 Mersilene suture, and reflected distally. Both heads of the rectus femoris are divided at their origin and reflected. The iliopsoas tendon is lengthened by transverse incisions, and the Pemberton iliac osteotomy lengthens the pelvis. Division of the psoas tendon (not the iliacus muscle) decreases the pressure over the femoral head.

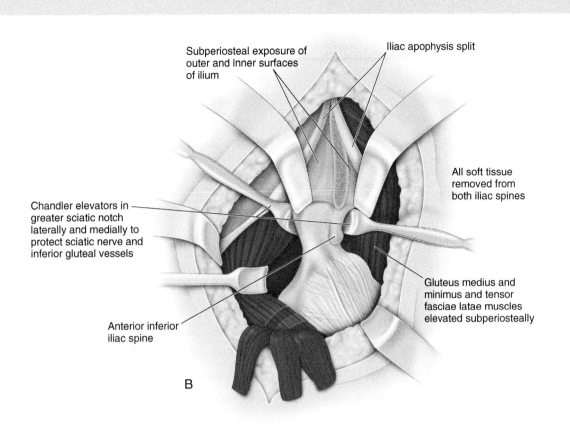

Subperiosteal exposure of outer and Inner surfaces of ilium

Iliac apophysis split

All soft tissue removed from both iliac spines

Chandler elevators in greater sciatic notch laterally and medially to protect sciatic nerve and inferior gluteal vessels

Gluteus medius and minimus and tensor fasciae latae muscles elevated subperiosteally

Anterior inferior iliac spine

B

B, The ilium is exposed subperiosteally all the way posteriorly. The interval between the greater sciatic notch and the hip joint capsule posteriorly is developed gently and cautiously. The periosteal elevator meets resistance at the posterior limb of the triradiate cartilage. Chandler elevator retractors are placed in the greater sciatic notch medially and laterally to protect the sciatic nerve and the gluteal vessels and nerves. On the inner wall of the pelvis, the periosteum and the cartilaginous apophysis may be divided anteriorly to posteriorly at the level of the anterior inferior iliac spine as far as the sciatic notch; this will facilitate the opening up of the osteotomy.

Continued on following page

Procedure 10   Pemberton Osteotomy, cont'd

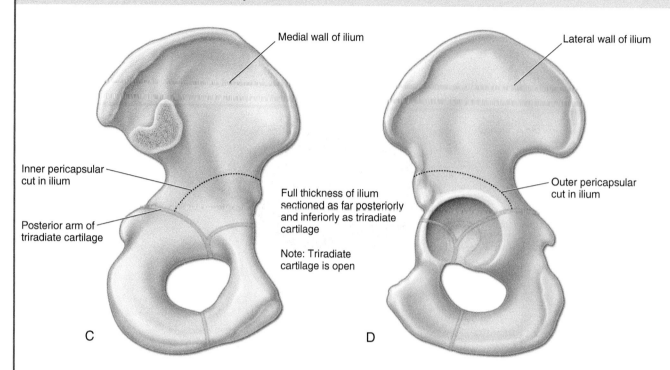

Medial wall of ilium

Lateral wall of ilium

Inner pericapsular cut in ilium

Outer pericapsular cut in ilium

Posterior arm of triradiate cartilage

Full thickness of ilium sectioned as far posteriorly and inferiorly as triradiate cartilage

Note: Triradiate cartilage is open

C

D

C to E, The osteotomy is first performed on the outer table of the ilium. The cut is curvilinear, and it describes a semicircle around the hip joint on the lateral side at a level that is 1 cm above the joint, between the anterior superior and anterior inferior iliac spines. It is best to mark the line of the osteotomy with indelible ink. The sharp edge of a thin osteotome is used to make the cut. The osteotomy ends at the posterior arm of the triradiate cartilage; this is most difficult to see if the exposure is inadequate. Image-intensification fluoroscopy helps to determine the terminal point of the cut at the triradiate cartilage, which is anterior to the greater sciatic notch and posterior to the hip joint margin. The next cut is made on the inner wall of the ilium, and it should be inferior to the level of the outer cut. The more distal the level of the inferior cut, the greater the extent of lateral coverage. If more anterior than superior coverage is required, then the medial and lateral cuts in the ilium are parallel. The importance of sectioning the ilium as far posterior and inferior to the triradiate cartilage as possible cannot be overemphasized. It is vital to not violate the articular cartilage of the acetabulum and enter the hip joint.

F, With sharp curved osteotomes, the cuts of the inner and outer table of the ilium are joined. Periosteal elevators are used to mobilize the osteotomized fragments, and the inferior segment of the ilium is leveled laterally, anteriorly, and distally.

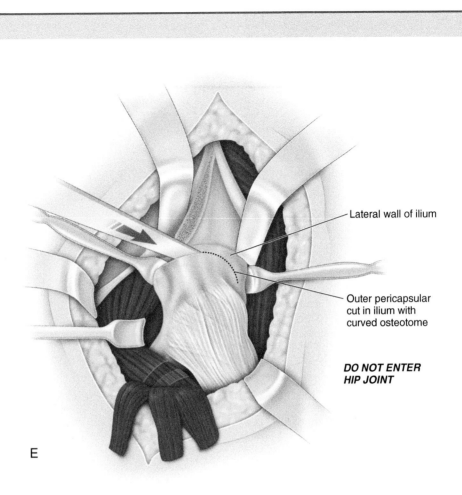

Lateral wall of ilium

Outer pericapsular
cut in ilium with
curved osteotome

***DO NOT ENTER
HIP JOINT***

E

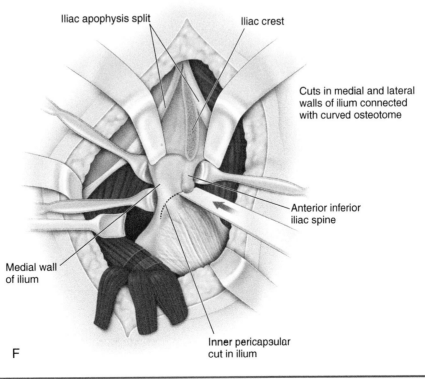

Iliac apophysis split

Iliac crest

Cuts in medial and lateral
walls of ilium connected
with curved osteotome

Anterior inferior
iliac spine

Medial wall
of ilium

Inner pericapsular
cut in ilium

F

Continued on following page

Procedure 10   Pemberton Osteotomy, cont'd

G, If necessary, a lamina spreader may be used to separate the iliac fragments. However, the operator should be very gentle; he or she should steady the upper segment of the ilium and push it distally. Care should be taken not to fracture the acetabular segment by forceful manipulation or crushing with the lamina spreader.

H and I, Next, a triangular wedge of bone is resected from the anterior part of the iliac wing. In the young child, we remove the wedge of bone more posteriorly and avoid the anterior superior iliac spine; this gives greater stability to the iliac fragments. The wedge of bone graft may be shaped into a curve to fit the graft site. Pemberton and Coleman recommend that grooves be made on the opposing cancellous surfaces of the osteotomy. The graft is impacted into the grooves, and the osteotomized fragment is sufficiently stable to obviate internal fixation. We do not recommend cutting grooves because of the associated problems of splintering and the weakening of the acetabulum. The fragments are fixed internally with two threaded Kirschner pins or cancellous screws. The internal fixation allows the surgeon to remove the cast sooner, to mobilize the hip, and to prevent joint stiffness. The sartorius muscle is reattached to its origin, the split iliac apophysis is sutured, and the wound is closed in the usual fashion. A one-and-one-half-hip spica cast is applied.

Postoperative Care

The cast is removed after 6 weeks, and the healing of the osteotomy is assessed with the use of anteroposterior and oblique lateral radiographs. When joint motion and the motor strength of the hip extensors, quadriceps, and triceps surae muscles are good, the child is allowed to ambulate. In the older patient, a three-point crutch gait with toe touch on the limb that was operated on is used to protect the hip until the Trendelenburg test is negative.

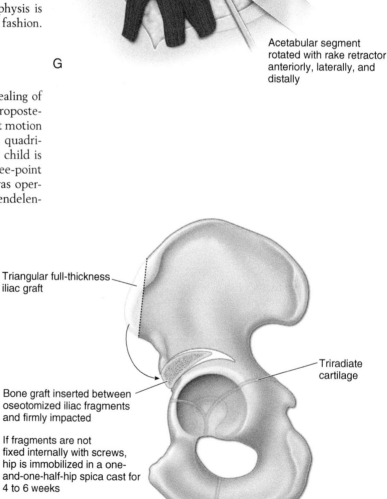

Upper segment of ilium held steady and pushed distally

Lamina spreader

Acetabular segment rotated with rake retractor anteriorly, laterally, and distally

G

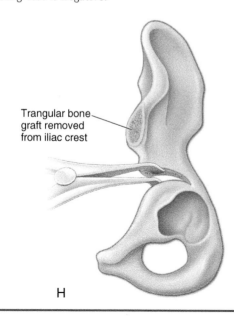

Trangular bone graft removed from iliac crest

H

Triangular full-thickness iliac graft

Triradiate cartilage

Bone graft inserted between oseotomized iliac fragments and firmly impacted

If fragments are not fixed internally with screws, hip is immobilized in a one-and-one-half-hip spica cast for 4 to 6 weeks

I

Procedure 11 Salter Innominate Osteotomy (see Video 5)

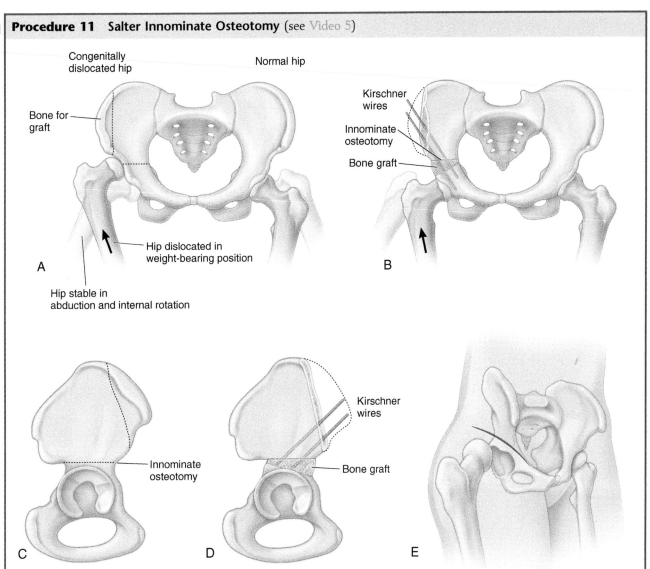

A, Congenitally dislocated hip — Normal hip — Bone for graft — Hip dislocated in weight-bearing position — Hip stable in abduction and internal rotation

B, Kirschner wires — Innominate osteotomy — Bone graft

C, Innominate osteotomy

D, Kirschner wires — Bone graft

E

Operative Technique

A to D, The Salter innominate osteotomy is based on the redirection of the acetabulum as a unit by hinging and rotation through the symphysis pubis, which is mobile in children. It is performed by making a transverse linear cut above the acetabulum at the level of the greater sciatic notch and the anterior inferior iliac spine. The whole acetabulum with the distal fragment of the innominate bone is tilted downward and laterally by rotating it. The new position of the distal fragment is maintained by a triangular bone graft that is taken from the proximal portion of the ilium and inserted into the open-wedge osteotomy site. Internal fixation is provided by two threaded Kirschner wires. Through the rotation and redirection of the acetabulum, the femoral head is covered adequately with the hip in a normal weight-bearing position. In other words, the reduced dislocation or subluxation that was previously stable in the position of flexion and abduction is now stable in the extended and neutral position of weight bearing.

E, The skin is prepared with the patient in the side-lying position so that the abdomen, the lower part of the chest, and the affected half of the pelvis can be draped to the midline anteriorly and posteriorly; the entire lower limb is also prepared and draped to allow for the free motion of the hip during the operation. The patient is placed supine with a roll beneath the buttock.

The skin incision is an oblique bikini incision. The incision that was formerly used over the iliac crest produces an unsightly scar, whereas the bikini incision results in excellent exposure and cosmesis. The anterior inferior iliac spine is palpated and marked. The incision begins approximately two thirds of the distance from the greater trochanter to the iliac crest and extends across the inferior spine and 1 or 2 cm beyond the inferior spine. The incision is then retracted over the iliac crest, and the dissection is carried down to the apophysis of the crest. Anteriorly, the tensor–sartorius interval is bluntly dissected, beginning distally and working proximally. The lateral femoral cutaneous nerve appears just medial to this interval and just distal to the inferior iliac spine, and it should be protected.

Continued on following page

Procedure 11   Salter Innominate Osteotomy, cont'd

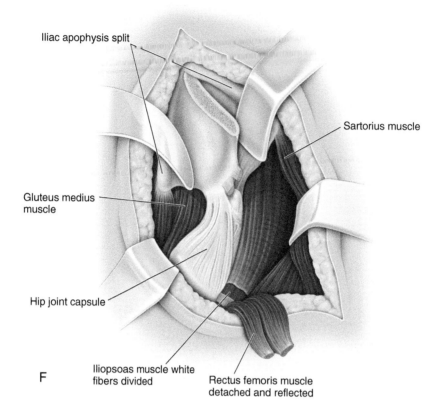

Iliac apophysis split

Sartorius muscle

Gluteus medius
muscle

Hip joint capsule

F

Iliopsoas muscle white
fibers divided

Rectus femoris muscle
detached and reflected

F, With a scalpel, the cartilaginous iliac apophysis is split in the middle down to the bone from the junction of its posterior and middle thirds to the anterior superior iliac spine. With the use of blunt dissection, the groove between the tensor fasciae latae and the sartorius and rectus femoris muscles is opened and developed. With a broad and long-handled periosteal elevator, the surgeon strips the lateral part of the iliac apophysis and the tensor fasciae latae and gluteus medius and minimus muscles subperiosteally and the greater sciatic notch posteromedially.

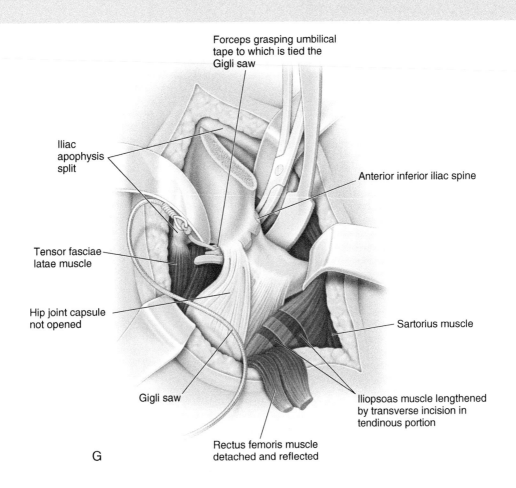

Forceps grasping umbilical
tape to which is tied the
Gigli saw

Iliac
apophysis
split

Anterior inferior iliac spine

Tensor fasciae
latae muscle

Hip joint capsule
not opened

Sartorius muscle

Gigli saw

Iliopsoas muscle lengthened
by transverse incision in
tendinous portion

Rectus femoris muscle
detached and reflected

G

G, Next, the periosteum is elevated from the medial and lateral walls of the ilium all the way posteriorly to the sciatic notch. It is vital to stay within the periosteum to prevent injury to the superior gluteal vessels and the sciatic nerve. A common pitfall is the inadequate surgical exposure of the sciatic notch, which makes it difficult to pass the Gigli saw behind the notch. The space on the lateral wall of the ilium is packed with sponge to dilate the interval and to control the oozing of blood. The periosteum is then elevated from the inner wall of the ilium in a continuous sheet to expose the sciatic notch medially. Again, it is important to stay in the subperiosteal plane to avoid injury to the vessels and nerves. The medial space is packed with sponge. The sartorius muscle can usually be reflected medially with the medial half of the cartilaginous iliac apophysis. If it is difficult to do so or if more distal exposure is desired, the origin of the sartorius muscle is detached from the anterior superior iliac spine, its free end is marked with whip sutures for later reattachment, and the muscle is reflected distally and medially. The two heads of origin of the rectus femoris—the direct one from the anterior inferior iliac spine and the reflected one from the superior margin of the acetabulum—are divided at their origin, marked with whip sutures, and reflected distally.

Next, on the deep surface of the iliopsoas muscle, the psoas tendon is exposed at the level of the pelvic rim.

The iliopsoas muscle is rolled over so that its tendinous portion can be separated from the muscular portion. If identification is in doubt, a nerve stimulator is used to distinguish the psoas tendon from the femoral nerve. A Freer elevator is passed between the tendinous and muscular portions of the iliopsoas muscle, and the psoas tendon is sectioned at one or two levels. The divided edges of the tendinous portion retract, and the muscle fibers separate, thus releasing the contractures of the iliopsoas without disturbing the continuity of the muscle.

Two medium-sized Hohmann elevator retractors—one introduced from the lateral side and the other from the medial side of the ilium—are placed subperiosteally in the sciatic notch. This step is crucial: in addition to keeping the neurovascular structures out of harm's way, the Hohmann retractors maintain the continuity of the proximal and distal innominate segments at the sciatic notch.

A right-angle forceps is passed subperiosteally from the medial side of the ilium and guided through the sciatic notch to the outer side with the index finger of the surgeon's opposite hand. The Gigli saw is most easily passed by first passing an umbilical tape through the notch. The end of the tape is tied to the Gigli saw. The tape is grasped with the right-angle clamp and pulled through the notch; it in turn pulls the saw through the notch.

Continued on following page

Procedure 11 Salter Innominate Osteotomy, cont'd

H, The osteotomy line extends from the sciatic notch to the anterior inferior iliac spine, and it is perpendicular to the sides of the ilium. It is vital to begin the osteotomy well inferiorly in the sciatic notch; the tendency is to start too high. The handles of the Gigli saw are kept widely separated and in continuous tension to keep the saw from binding in the soft cancellous bone. The osteotomy, which emerges anteriorly immediately above the anterior inferior iliac spine, is completed with the Gigli saw. The use of an osteotome may subject the superior gluteal artery and the sciatic nerve to iatrogenic damage. **I,** The Hohmann retractors are kept constantly at the sciatic notch by an assistant to prevent the posterior or medial displacement of the distal segment and the loss of bony continuity posteriorly. A triangular full-thickness bone graft is removed from the anterior part of the iliac crest with a large, straight, double-action bone cutter. The length of the base of the triangular wedge represents the distance between the anterior superior iliac spine and the anterior inferior iliac spine. The portion of bone to be removed as a bone graft is held firmly with a Kocher forceps; the operator must be sure that this portion does not fall on the floor or get contaminated.

The proximal fragment of the innominate bone is held steady with a large towel-clip forceps, and the distal fragment is grasped with a second stout towel forceps. The affected hip is placed in 90 degrees of flexion, maximal abduction, and 90 degrees of lateral rotation; a second assistant applies distal and lateral traction to the thigh. With the second towel clip placed well posteriorly on the distal fragment, the surgeon rotates the distal fragment downward, outward, and forward, thereby opening the osteotomy site anteriorly. The site must be kept closed posteriorly. Leaving it open posteriorly displaces the hip joint distally without adequate rotation and redirection of the acetabulum at the symphysis pubis; furthermore, it will lengthen the lower limb unnecessarily. Another technical error to avoid is opening the osteotomy site with a mechanical spreader (e.g., a laminectomy spreader, a self-retaining retractor) because that may move the proximal fragment upward and the distal fragment downward without rotating the distal fragment through the symphysis pubis. The acetabular maldirection will not be corrected unless such rotation of the distal fragment takes place. The posterior and medial displacement of the distal fragment should be avoided.

When the periosteum on the median wall of the ilium is taut, the cartilaginous apophysis of the ilium is divided at two or three levels; this will help with the rotation of the acetabulum.

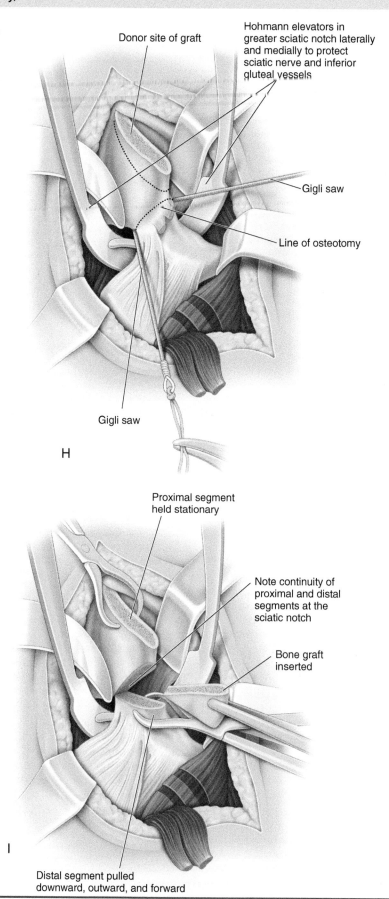

Donor site of graft

Hohmann elevators in greater sciatic notch laterally and medially to protect sciatic nerve and inferior gluteal vessels

Gigli saw

Line of osteotomy

Gigli saw

H

Proximal segment held stationary

Note continuity of proximal and distal segments at the sciatic notch

Bone graft inserted

I

Distal segment pulled downward, outward, and forward

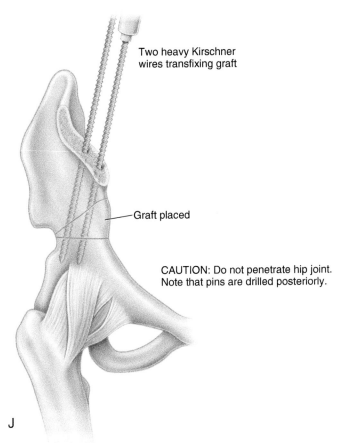

Two heavy Kirschner
wires transfixing graft

Graft placed

CAUTION: Do not penetrate hip joint.
Note that pins are drilled posteriorly.

J

J, Next, the bone graft is shaped with bone cutters to the appropriate size to fit the open osteotomy site. The graft is usually about the correct size for the size of the patient because the base of the triangular graft represents the distance between the anterior superior iliac spine and the anterior inferior iliac spine. The surgeon should avoid using a large graft and hammering it in to fit snugly into the osteotomy site because this will open the site posteriorly. With the osteotomy site open anteriorly and the distal segment rotated, the bone graft is inserted into the opened-up osteotomy. The distal fragment of the innominate bone should be kept slightly anterior to the proximal fragment. When traction is released, the graft is firmly locked by the two segments of the bone.

A stout threaded Kirschner wire is drilled from the proximal segment across the osteotomy site, through the graft, and into the distal segment posterior to the acetabulum, thereby preventing any future displacement of the graft or the distal segment. The first wire should be directed posterior to the acetabulum. Radiographs are obtained to check the adequacy of correction of the acetabular maldirection and the position of the Kirschner wire. A second Kirschner wire is then drilled parallel to the first to further stabilize the internal fixation of the osteotomy. In the older child, we use a third threaded Kirschner wire or two cancellous positional screws to ensure the security of internal fixation. The inadequate penetration of the wires into the distal fragment will result in the loss of alignment of the osteotomy. The wires may bend or break, or, if they are excessively heavy, they may fracture the graft or the innominate bone; the importance of choosing the correct diameter of wire or cancellous screw cannot be overemphasized. The penetration of the wires into the hip joint may cause chondrolysis of the hip, or it may cause the wire to break at the joint level. An anteroposterior radiograph of the hips is obtained to check the depth of the Kirschner wires and the degree of correction that has been obtained.

The two halves of the cartilaginous iliac apophysis are sutured together over the iliac crest. The rectus femoris and sartorius muscles are reattached to their origins, and the wound is closed in a routine manner. Skin closure should be with continuous subcuticular 00 nylon suture. The Kirschner wires are cut so that their ends are in the subcutaneous fat and easily palpable.

A one-and-one-half-hip spica cast is applied with the hip in a stable weight-bearing position. Immobilization in a forced or extreme position should be avoided because it will cause the excessive and continuous compression of articular cartilage, osteonecrosis, permanent joint stiffness, and eventual degenerative arthritis. In the cast, the knee is bent to control the position of hip rotation. When there is excessive femoral antetorsion, the hip is immobilized in slight medial rotation. A common pitfall is immobilization in marked medial rotation; this mistake will result in posterior subluxation or dislocation of the femoral head. With femoral retrotorsion, the hip should be immobilized in slight lateral rotation.

A radiograph of the hips through the cast is obtained before the child is discharged from the hospital. Another set of radiographs is obtained 2 to 3 weeks after surgery to ensure that the graft has not collapsed, that the pins have not migrated, and that there is no medial displacement of the distal segments. In the older cooperative patient, when cancellous screws are used for internal fixation, a hip spica cast is not necessary.

Postoperative Care

The cast is removed after 6 weeks with the child under general anesthesia, and the pins are removed through a portion of the original incision. Range-of-motion exercises are begun, and the patient is allowed to ambulate with support. Older children can use crutches; those who are younger than 5 years old use a walker. Full weight bearing is resumed after 3 weeks if the range of motion of the knee is more than 90 degrees. When an open reduction has been combined with a Salter osteotomy, a second period of immobilization in abduction casts (Petrie casts) for approximately 4 weeks is recommended. This allows the hips to regain flexion and extension, and the abducted position maintains hip reduction.

Procedure 12 Ganz Periacetabular Osteotomy

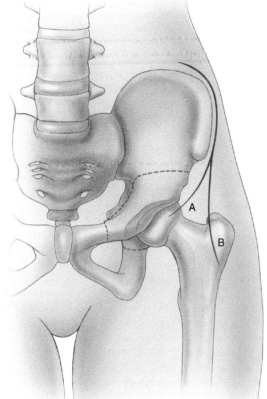

A

Operative Technique

A, Two types of incisions can be made. Both incisions track along the iliac crest until ending just over the anterior superior iliac spine (ASIS). *A,* The incision continues medially and distally and is used for the more straightforward PAO when previous surgery has not occurred and looking in the hip joint is not planned. *B,* The incision curves distally and laterally over an imaginary area over the tensor fascia lata and is used for more challenging hips and/or when an arthrotomy is planned. **B,** The fascia of the tensor fascia lata is incised, and the muscle is retracted laterally and the fascia medially. The sartorius and the fascia from the tensor fascia are retracted medially with the osteotomized anterior superior iliac spin. **C,** Ischial osteotomy. A soft tissue dissection is made between the direct head of the rectus muscle and the iliacus-ilicapsularis-iliopsoas muscle. Capsular exposure. The ilicapsularis muscle is sharply dissected off the capsule. **D,** A curved Mayo retractor is placed between the capsule and the psoas opening a window to allow the osteotome to enter. **E,** The ishial osteotomy is made beginning below the acetabulum and directed posteriorly under fluoroscopy using the AP and the false profile projections.

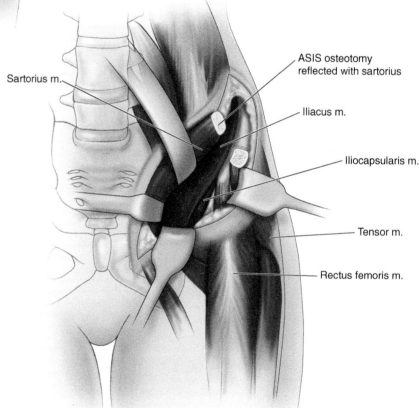

Sartorius m.

ASIS osteotomy reflected with sartorius

Iliacus m.

Iliocapsularis m.

Tensor m.

Rectus femoris m.

B

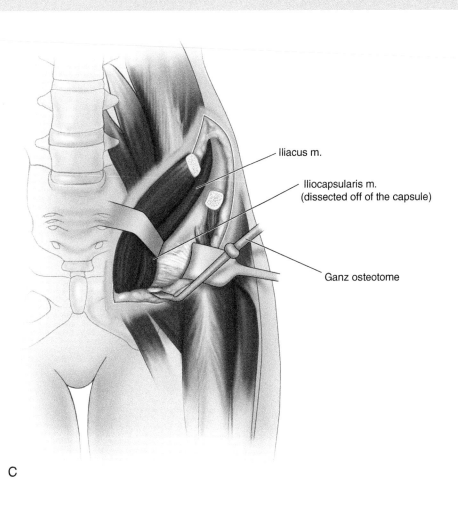

Iliacus m.

Iliocapsularis m.
(dissected off of the capsule)

Ganz osteotome

C

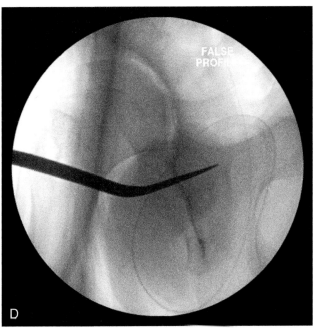

D

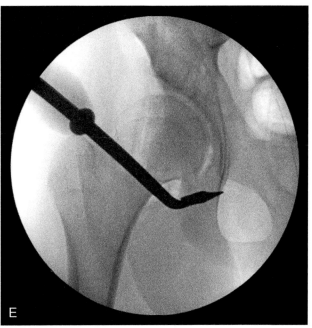

E

Continued on following page

Procedure 12   Ganz Periacetabular Osteotomy, cont'd

F, The Superior ramus osteotomy. Soft tissue dissection first elevates the ileopectineal fascia over the pelvic brim and into the obturator foramen, and soft tissue retractors are placed circumferentially into the obturator. A sharp-tipped Homan is placed on the anterior aspect of the superior ramus. A straight osteotomy begins the osteotomy just medial to the ileopectineal eminence and is directed at 45 degrees from the horizontal to maintain a floor for the ileopsoas tendon. G, The innominate osteotomy. A small soft tissue window is made on the lateral aspect of the iliac wing and a smooth Homan is placed to protect the muscle. The osteotomy begins at the tip of the anterior superior iliac spine and is directed down to the floor ending just lateral to the pelvic brim. A fluoroscopic false profile image should be made to ensure this endpoint will allow for an adequate posterior column osteotomy. H, The posterior column osteotomy. A long-curved osteotomy with a rotation-controlling handle is used to make this cut. I, The false profile radiograph is used to ensure this cut is posterior to the acetabulum but anterior to the posterior edge of the posterior column.

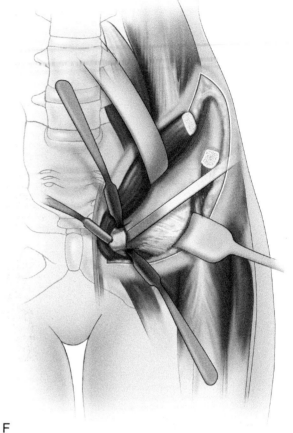

F

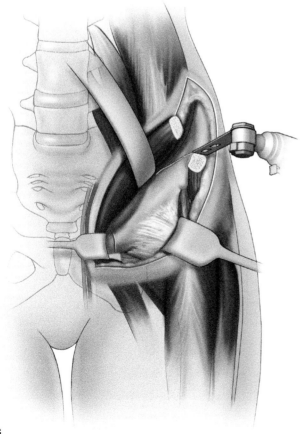

G

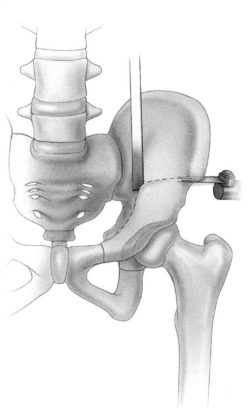

H

Manipulation and positioning of the acetabular fragment. **J,** A Shanz pin is placed just superior to the acetabulum. First, the fragment is positioned by disengaging the superior ramus to allow for medicalization of the hip joint center and to ensure adequate restoration or maintenance of version. The primary correction maneuver is forward rotation with slight tipping of the fragment medially. The radiographs should demonstrate four key points: 1. Lateral coverage; 2. Anterior coverage; 3. Medicalization; and 4. Normal version. **K,** This fluoroscopic view demonstrates overcorrection with excess medicalization and lateral coverage with a downturning sourcil. **L,** Following repositioning, the sourcil is horizontal with good lateral coverage, normal version, and normal medicalization with restoration of Shenton's line.

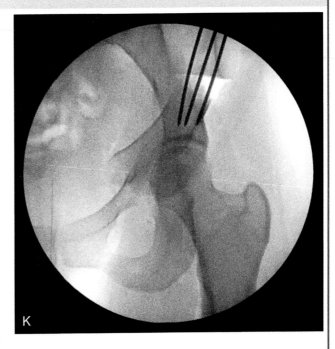

K

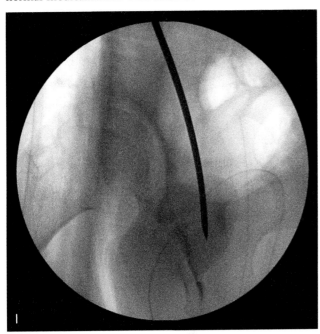

I

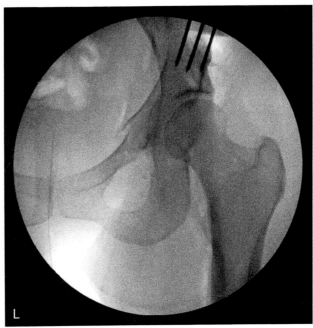

L

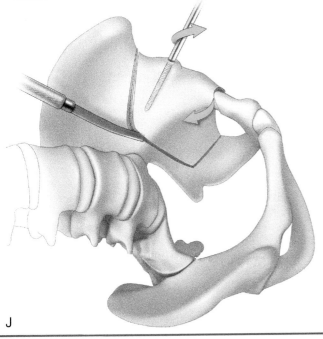

J

Procedure 13   Percutaneous Cannulated Screw Fixation ("Pinning") of Slipped Capital Femoral Epiphysis

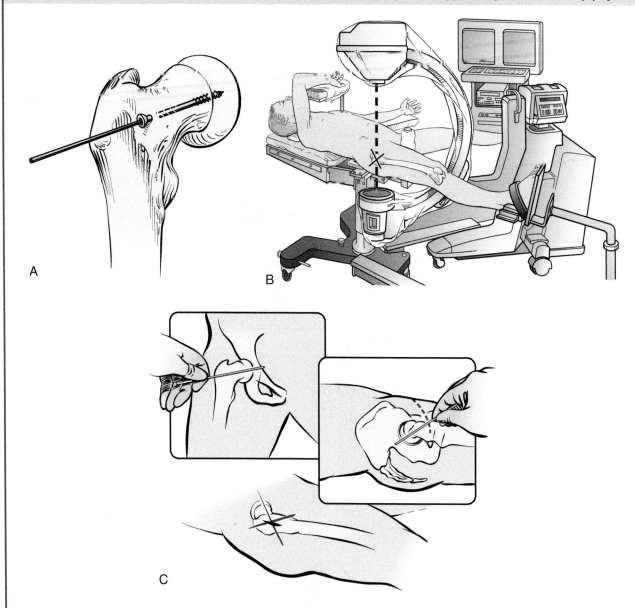

A

B

C

A, The ideal position of a single cannulated screw is in the center of the epiphysis, perpendicular to the physis. In this position, stabilization of the epiphysis to the neck is maximal and the risk is lowest for inadvertent penetration of the screw into the joint. Because of the typical posterior displacement of the femoral epiphysis on the neck, the guidewire and screw must be located on the anterior base of the femoral neck in most cases. The exact location varies with the severity of the slip.

B, The patient is positioned on the fracture table with the patella facing anteriorly and the limb in neutral to slight abduction. In the case of unstable slips, the epiphysis will usually be noted to have reduced to some extent in this position. No further efforts at reduction should be made.

The opposite limb can be placed in traction and maximum abduction, or flexed and abducted to clear it from the lateral fluoroscopic projection. Proper functioning of the fluoroscope with adequate anteroposterior (AP) and lateral visualization of the femoral epiphysis should be confirmed at this time. The C-arm fluoroscope is then draped out of the surgical field.

C, The ideal trajectory is identified and marked on the patient's skin by placing a free guidewire against the skin while assessing the position of the guidewire under fluoroscopy on both the AP and lateral projections. The intersection of these two lines indicates the proper point of insertion of the guidewire into the patient's limb. A stab incision in the skin is made at this point.

D, Under fluoroscopic guidance, and following the trajectories marked on the patient's skin, the guidewire is pushed onto the base of the femoral neck, then advanced into the neck, across the physis, and into the epiphysis. If the location of the guidewire is not ideal, it should be repositioned, or temporarily left in place as a guide for the insertion of a second guidewire in the proper position. Great care must be exercised that the guidewire (and subsequently the drill, tap, and screw) is not advanced into the hip joint. For unstable slips, a second guidewire is inserted parallel to the first, preferably into the inferomedial quadrant of the epiphysis. This provides some rotational stability in the case of unstable slips and can be used for the insertion of a second cannulated screw if desired.

E, The length of guidewire inserted into the bone is measured either with the cannulated depth gauge instrument (a) or by placing a second guidewire against the femoral neck parallel to that in the femur and measuring the difference of exposed ends of the guidewire. The femoral neck and epiphysis are then drilled and tapped using the cannulated instruments. The cannulated drill is advanced over the guidewire (b), and the screw is inserted over the guidewire. The position of the guidewire is checked periodically to make sure it is not being inadvertently advanced into the hip or withdrawn from the femur with the drill or tap.

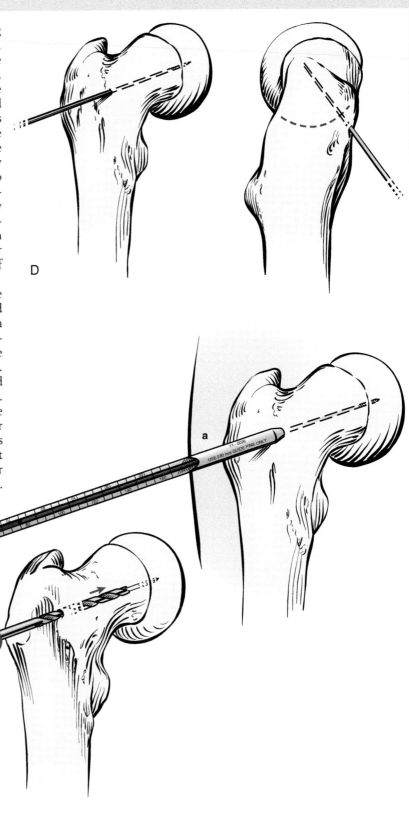

Continued on following page

Procedure 13 Percutaneous Cannulated Screw Fixation ("Pinning") of Slipped Capital Femoral Epiphysis, cont'd

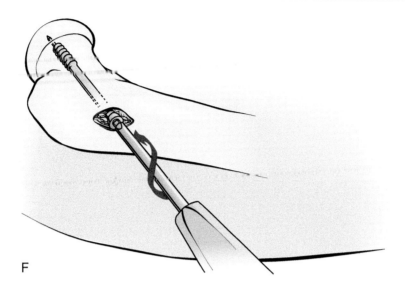

F

F, A screw of proper length is inserted across the physis into the epiphysis. We prefer to have threads cross the physis, and we do not try to achieve compression between the femoral cortex and the threads of the screw. The screw head should not be left protruding through the femoral cortex more than a few millimeters or it may irritate the soft tissues and cause symptoms. In the case of unstable slips, a second screw may be inserted. The guidewire is withdrawn. Careful assessment should be made before closing the skin to ensure that the screw does not penetrate the joint. The incision can be closed with one or two absorbable subcutaneous and skin sutures.

Postoperative Management

The patient is taught to use crutches as soon as comfortable. We allow patients with stable slips to bear weight as tolerated, and those with unstable slips to bear partial weight for 6 weeks. The patient is subsequently periodically reexamined with radiographs to confirm physeal closure and to monitor the contralateral hip until skeletal maturity.

Procedure 14   Scheme and Principles of the Dunn Procedure (Open Reduction of the Capital Epiphysis With Shortening of the Femoral Neck)

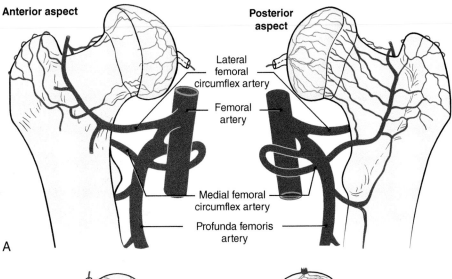

Anterior aspect

Posterior aspect

Lateral femoral circumflex artery

Femoral artery

Medial femoral circumflex artery

Profunda femoris artery

A

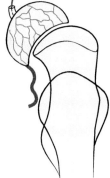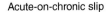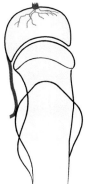

Acute-on-chronic slip

Retinacular vessels shorten after a few days

Attempted closed reduction will stretch blood vessels

Only blood supply to head is from artery of ligamentum teres

B

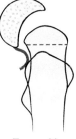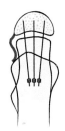

Trapezoid osteotomy of neck

Neck shortened

Retinacular vessels relaxed

C

A, A schematic representation showing the blood supply to the capital epiphysis. The predominant system is the medial circumflex artery and the lateral epiphyseal system, with a variable and relatively minor supply from the ligamentum teres and perforating metaphyseal vessels.
B, With posterior slipping of the capital epiphysis, the posterior periosteum is stripped away from the femoral neck, along with the epiphyseal blood supply. The vessels likely shorten in this position. The vessels may be damaged by any attempt to reduce the epiphysis (open or closed) with the vessels in this shortened condition.
C, By resecting the callus and posterior "beak" and carefully preserving the vessels from direct injury, the operator can reduce the epiphysis and fix it to the femoral neck without stretching the vessels.

Procedure 15 Intraarticular Hip Fusion for Avascular Necrosis

A, The patient is positioned on a radiolucent tabletop with the entire affected lower extremity draped free and with C-arm fluoroscopy available. An anterior approach to the hip is best with this technique, exposing the anterior femoral capsule and subsequently the inner aspect of the ilium for insertion of the screws across the ilium into the femoral head and neck. *I,* Iliac muscle (m.); *Ps,* psoas major m.; *RF,* rectus femoris m.; *S,* sartorius m.; *TFL,* tensor fasciae latae m.; *VL,* vastus lateralis m.; *VM,* vastus medialis m.

B, The anterior capsule of the hip is exposed broadly through this approach. The iliac muscle is also stripped from the inner wall of the pelvis.

C, The femoral head is exposed and dislocated from the acetabulum. Necrotic bone is removed from the femoral head with rongeurs and cup arthroplasty reamers. The acetabulum is similarly prepared with curets and cup arthroplasty reamers, removing all articular cartilage and sclerotic bone.

D, The denuded femoral head is reduced into the acetabulum into a "best fit" position. One or two cannulated screws are then inserted from the inner wall of the pelvis across the joint into the femoral head and neck. Fluoroscopic visualization may be required for optimum insertion and control of the depth of insertion into the femoral neck.

E, An intertrochanteric or subtrochanteric osteotomy is made to allow repositioning of the leg in a position of slight abduction and external rotation. Normally the leg should be placed in a position of extension in the supine position. The upper femur may be exposed through a separate lateral incision, or by extending the anterior exposure and reflecting the vastus lateralis from the anterior aspect of the femur. If the osteotomy is unstable, an intramedullary rod (e.g., a Rush rod) may be inserted into the medullary canal for partial control of the femoral fragments.

Postoperative Management

The patient is placed in a one-and-one-half-hip spica cast until union of the fusion and femoral osteotomy. Alternatively, external fixation of the pelvis to the lower femoral fragment may be used.

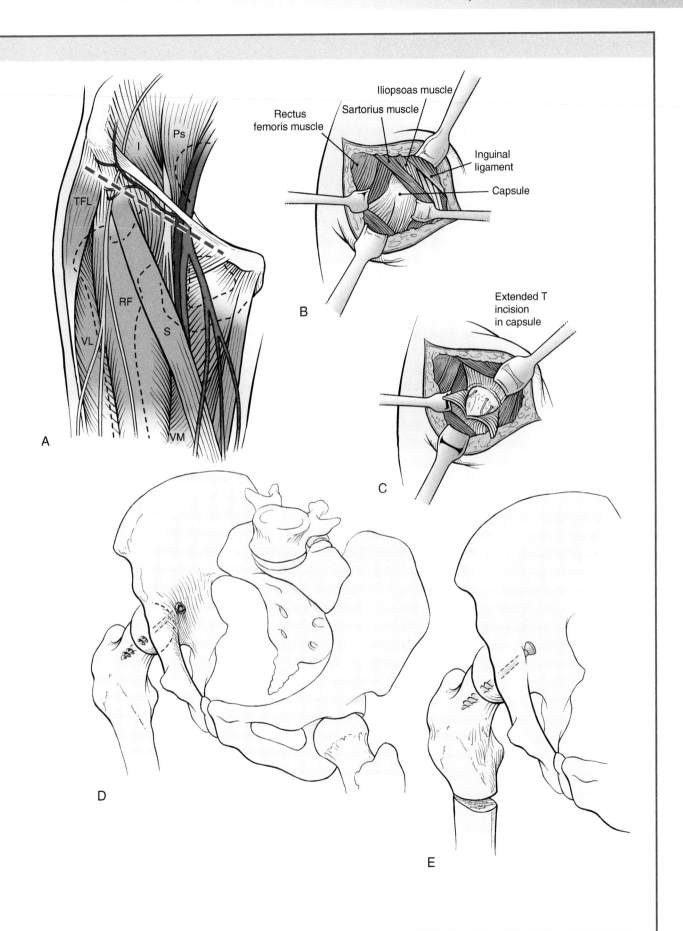

Procedure 16   Pauwels' Intertrochanteric Y-Osteotomy

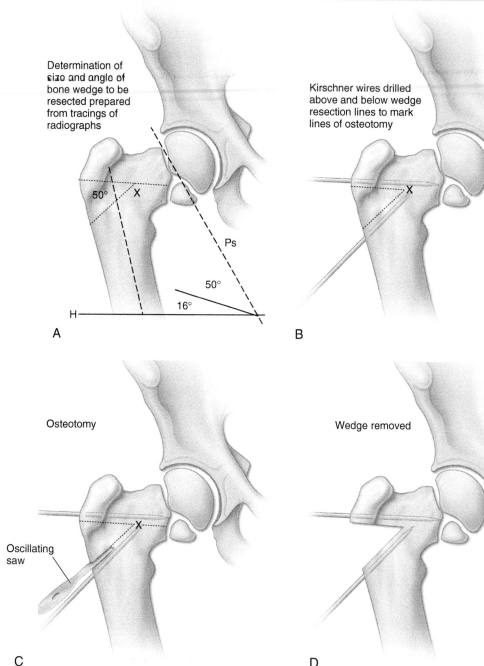

Determination of size and angle of bone wedge to be resected prepared from tracings of radiographs

50°

X

Ps

50°

16°

H

A

Kirschner wires drilled above and below wedge resection lines to mark lines of osteotomy

X

B

Osteotomy

Oscillating saw

X

C

Wedge removed

D

The patient is placed supine on a radiolucent operating table. The hip and upper end of the femur should be clearly visualized on the image intensifier. The entire hip and lower limb are prepared and draped to allow free movement of the limb. The surgeon may prefer older children be placed on a fracture table. The upper end of the femur and trochanteric region are exposed through a direct lateral approach.

Operative Technique

A, The angle of bone wedge to be resected is determined from tracings of the preoperative radiograph.

B, Under image intensifier control, the lines of osteotomy are defined by drilling guiding Kirschner wires parallel to the intended bone cuts above and below the wedge resection lines. The upper Kirschner wire should stop short of the capital physis and the defect of the femoral neck, and the tip of the lower Kirschner wire should be just below the upper osteotomy line and terminate medial to point X (the apex of the wedge of bone to be resected). **C,** With an oscillating saw, the upper intertrochanteric osteotomy is performed, and the wedge of bone is resected. **D,** The wedge of bone is removed with flat osteotomes.

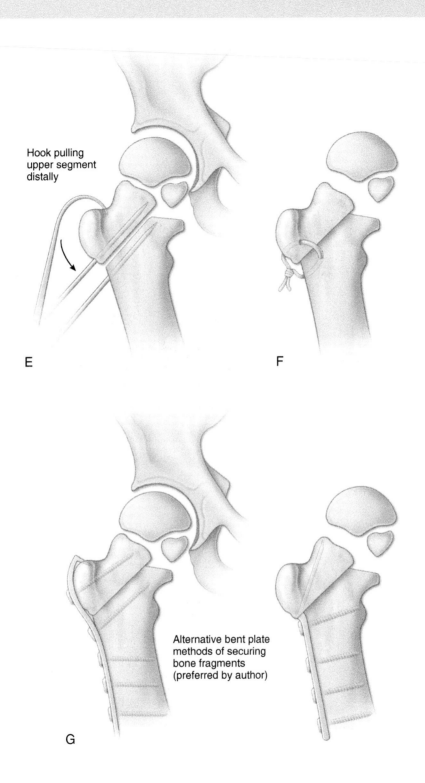

E, A hook over the greater trochanter is used to pull the upper segment distally, and the two Kirschner wires are made parallel to each other, to close the gap.

F, Pauwels recommended fixing the fragments with a tension band wire loop passed through drill holes in each fragment.

G, Preferable alternatives for internal fixation are to use either a contoured plate and screws over the greater trochanter to the distal fragment or a blade plate or sliding compression screw and plate fixation device.

Procedure 17   Hemipelvectomy (Banks and Coleman Technique)

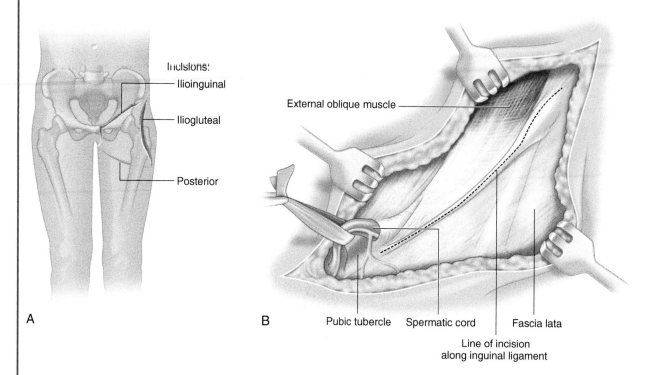

Incisions:
— Ilioinguinal
— Iliogluteal
— Posterior

A

External oblique muscle

B

Pubic tubercle   Spermatic cord   Fascia lata

Line of incision
along inguinal ligament

The patient lies on the unaffected side and is maintained in position with sandbags and kidney rests, which are placed well above the iliac crests. The normal limb underneath is flexed at the hip and knee and fastened to the table by wide adhesive straps. The uppermost arm is supported on a rest. The perineal area and, in the male, scrotum and penis, are shielded and held out of the operative field with sterile, self-adhering skin drapes. The operative area is prepared and draped so that the proximal thigh, inguinal and gluteal regions, and abdomen are sterile. It should be possible to turn the patient onto his or her back and side without contaminating the surgical field.

A, The outlines of the skin flaps, consisting of ilioinguinal, iliogluteal, and posterior incisions, are marked. With the patient placed on his or her back, the ilioinguinal incision is made first. It begins at the pubic tubercle and passes upward and backward parallel to Poupart ligament to the anterior superior iliac spine and then posteriorly on the iliac crest. Its posterior limit depends on the desired level of section of the innominate bone.

B, The subcutaneous tissue and fascia are divided along the line of the skin incision. The insertions of the abdominal muscles superiorly and the tensor fasciae latae and gluteus medius inferiorly are detached extraperiosteally from the iliac crest.

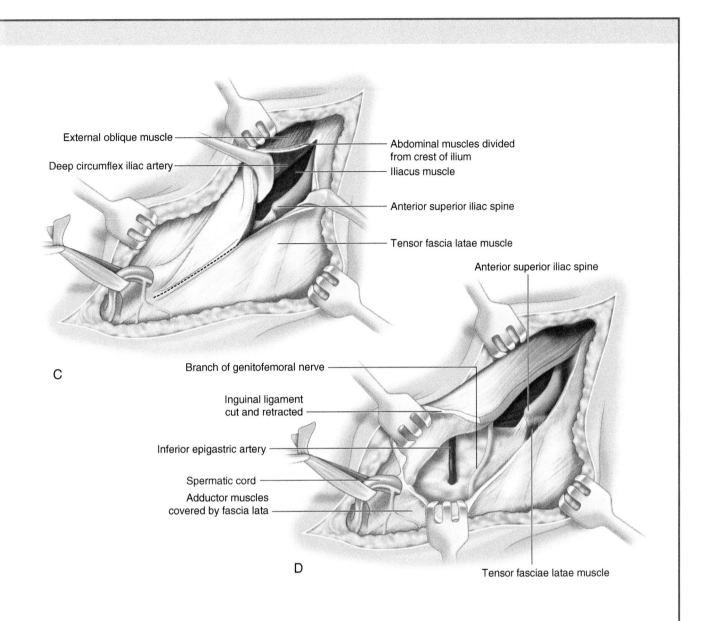

External oblique muscle

Deep circumflex iliac artery

Abdominal muscles divided
from crest of ilium

Iliacus muscle

Anterior superior iliac spine

Tensor fascia latae muscle

C

Anterior superior iliac spine

Branch of genitofemoral nerve

Inguinal ligament
cut and retracted

Inferior epigastric artery

Spermatic cord

Adductor muscles
covered by fascia lata

Tensor fasciae latae muscle

D

C, The abdominal muscles are detached from the iliac crest and medial wall of the ilium. The tributaries of the deep circumflex vessels are ligated.

D, The inguinal ligament is divided and retracted superiorly, along with the spermatic cord and abdominal muscles. The lower skin flap is retracted inferiorly, and the inner pelvis is freed by blunt dissection. The inferior epigastric artery and lumboinguinal nerve are exposed, ligated, and divided.

Continued on following page

Procedure 17   Hemipelvectomy (Banks and Coleman Technique), cont'd

Abdominal muscles
and inguinal ligament
divided and retracted

External iliac
vessels

Sheath opened

Lymph nodes

Femoral nerve

Inferior epigastric artery

Femoral vein

E

Bladder retracted
Rectus abdominis muscle
detached from pubic bone

External iliac artery and vein

Femoral nerve retracted (and divided
also for external hemipelvectomy)

Pubic bone exposed
subperiosteally

Superior ramus
of pubis

Spermatic cord retracted

Adductor muscle detached
from pubic bone
Line of osteotomy of pubic bone
(½ inch lateral to symphysis pubis)

F

E, In the loose areolar tissue, the external iliac vessels are dissected, and femoral nerve is divided and dissected. The external iliac artery and vein are individually clamped, severed, and doubly ligated with size 0 silk sutures.

F, The rectus abdominis and adductor muscles are detached from the pubic bone, which is extraperiosteally exposed. The bladder is retracted superiorly. The pubic bone is osteotomized 1.5 cm lateral to the symphysis. Depending on the proximity of the tumor, the osteotomy may have to be made at the symphysis pubis. Injury to the bladder or urethra should be avoided. Any bleeding from the retropubic venous plexus is controlled by coagulation and packing with warm laparotomy pads.

G, The patient is then turned onto her or his side. The drapes are adjusted and reinforced to ensure sterility of the operative field. First, the anterior incision is extended posteriorly to the posterior superior iliac spine. From the upper end of the anterior incision, the second or iliogluteal incision is started. It extends to the thigh, curving forward to an area approximately 5 cm distal to the greater trochanter. It then passes backward around the posterior aspect of the thigh to meet the anterior incision. The subcutaneous tissue and fascia are divided in line with the skin incision.

H, The sciatic nerve is clamped, ligated, and sharply divided distal to the origin of the inferior gluteal nerve. The piriformis, gemellus, and obturator internus muscles are transected near their insertion.

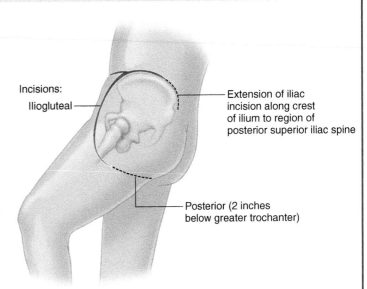

Incisions:
Iliogluteal

Extension of iliac incision along crest of ilium to region of posterior superior iliac spine

Posterior (2 inches below greater trochanter)

G

Transection to reflect gluteus medius muscle

Gluteus medius and minimus muscles

Line of transection of piriformis muscle

Line of transection of sciatic nerve

Obturator internus muscle and gemelli muscles

Greater trochanter

Quadratus femoris muscle

Vessels and nerves to gluteus maximus muscle are preserved

Superior gluteal artery

Inferior gluteal artery

Inferior gluteal nerve

Posterior cutaneous nerve of thigh

Semitendinosus muscle

Gluteus maximus muscle

H

Continued on following page

Procedure 17 Hemipelvectomy (Banks and Coleman Technique), cont'd

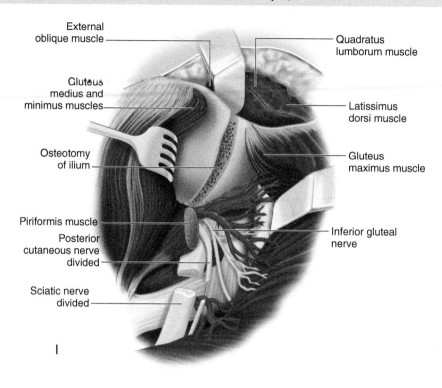

I

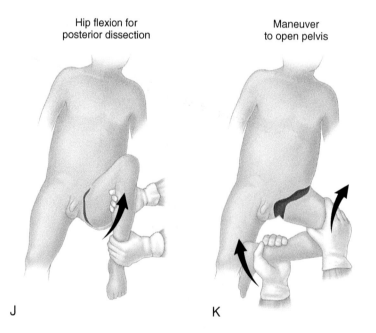

Hip flexion for
posterior dissection

Maneuver
to open pelvis

J   K

I, The ilium is exposed subperiosteally by elevation and detachment of the latissimus dorsi and sacrospinalis muscles, posterior portion of the gluteus medius, and anterior fibers of the gluteus maximus. The inner wall of the ilium is also exposed subperiosteally, anterior to the sacroiliac joint. Retractors are placed in the sciatic notch and, using a Gigli saw, the ilium is osteotomized approximately 5 cm anterior to the posterior gluteal line. The site of the ilium osteotomy depends on the location of the tumor; it is placed farther posteriorly if the neoplasm is adjacent to the gluteal line.

J, The patient is repositioned on his or her back, and the hip is maximally flexed in some abduction. The posterior incision is completed.

K, The hip is manipulated into maximal abduction and external rotation, laying open the pelvic area and widely exposing the remaining intrapelvic structures to be severed.

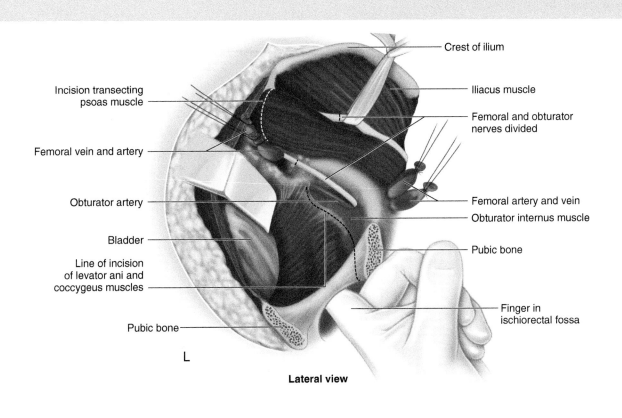

Crest of ilium

Incision transecting
psoas muscle

Iliacus muscle

Femoral and obturator
nerves divided

Femoral vein and artery

Obturator artery

Femoral artery and vein

Obturator internus muscle

Bladder

Pubic bone

Line of incision
of levator ani and
coccygeus muscles

Finger in
ischiorectal fossa

Pubic bone

L

Lateral view

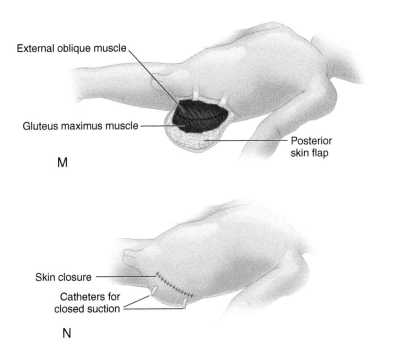

External oblique muscle

Gluteus maximus muscle

Posterior
skin flap

M

Skin closure

Catheters for
closed suction

N

L, From above downward, the femoral nerve, iliopsoas muscle, obturator vessels, obturator nerve, levator ani, and coccygeus muscles are sectioned. The vessels are doubly ligated before division to prevent troublesome bleeding.

M, The gluteus maximus muscle is sutured to the divided margin of the external oblique muscle and lateral abdominal wall. A couple of perforated silicone catheters are inserted and connected to closed-suction drainage.
N, Fascia, subcutaneous tissue, and skin are closed in layers in the usual manner. A pressure dressing is applied.

Procedure 18   Hip Disarticulation

Racquet-type incision

A

Sartorius muscle divided at origin

Gluteus medius muscle

Tensor fasciae latae muscle

Articular capsule

Vastus lateralis muscle

Vastus intermedius muscle

Vastus medialis muscle

Rectus femoris muscle reflected

Rectus femoris muscle divided at origins

Iliopsoas muscle

Femoral nerve ligated and divided over tongue blade

Pectineus muscle

Femoral artery and vein doubly ligated and divided

Adductor longus muscle

Gracilis muscle

Sartorius muscle reflected

B

A, An anterior racquet-type incision is made starting at the anterior superior iliac spine and extending medially and distally, parallel to Poupart ligament, to the middle of the inner aspect of the thigh, approximately 2 inches distal to the origin of the adductor muscles. It is then continued around the back of the thigh at a level approximately 2 inches distal to the ischial tuberosity. Next, the incision is carried along the lateral aspect of the thigh approximately 3 inches distal to the base of the greater trochanter and is curved proximally and medially to join the first incision at the anterior superior iliac spine.

B, The subcutaneous tissue and fascia are divided in line with the skin incision. The long saphenous vein is exposed and ligated after the operator traces it to its junction with the femoral vein. If lymph node dissection is indicated, it can be performed at this stage. The sartorius muscle is divided at its origin from the anterior superior iliac spine and reflected distally. The origins of the two heads of the rectus femoris—one from the anterior inferior iliac spine and the other from the superior margin of the acetabulum—are detached and reflected distally. The femoral nerve is isolated, ligated with size 0 silk sutures, and divided on a tongue blade with a sharp scalpel or razor blade just distal to the ligature. The femoral artery and vein are isolated, doubly ligated with size 0 silk sutures proximally and distally, and severed in between the sutures.

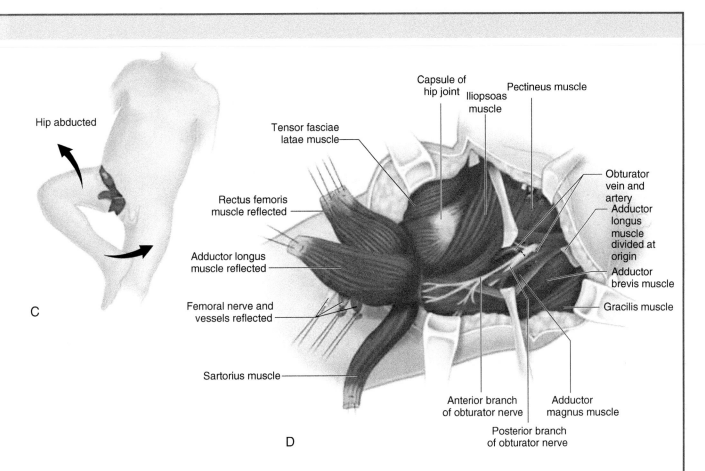

Hip abducted

C

Tensor fasciae
latae muscle

Rectus femoris
muscle reflected

Adductor longus
muscle reflected

Femoral nerve and
vessels reflected

Sartorius muscle

Capsule of
hip joint
Iliopsoas
muscle

Pectineus muscle

Obturator
vein and
artery
Adductor
longus
muscle
divided at
origin
Adductor
brevis muscle

Gracilis muscle

Anterior branch
of obturator nerve

Adductor
magnus muscle

Posterior branch
of obturator nerve

D

C, The hip is abducted to expose its medial aspect, and the adductor longus is detached at its origin from the pubis and reflected distally. The anterior branch of the obturator nerve is exposed deep to the adductor longus and traced proximally.

D, The adductor brevis is retracted posteriorly. The posterior branch of the obturator nerve is isolated and dissected proximal to the main trunk of the obturator nerve, which is sharply divided. Next, the obturator vessels are isolated and ligated. One should be careful not to sever the obturator artery inadvertently because it will retract into the pelvis and cause bleeding that is difficult to control.

Continued on following page

Procedure 18   Hip Disarticulation, cont'd

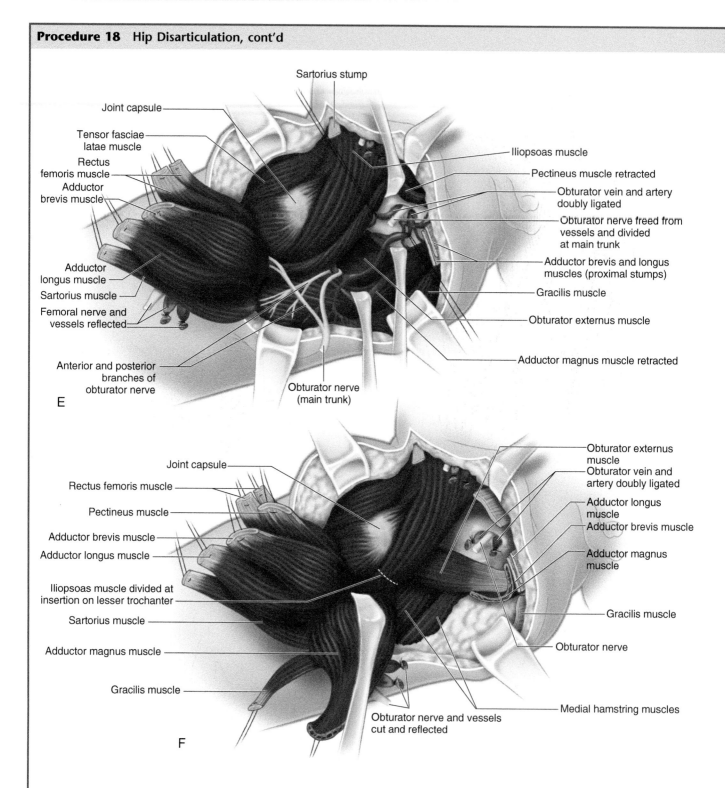

E, The pectineus, adductor brevis, gracilis, and adductor magnus are severed near their origins. It is best to use a coagulation knife.

F, The hip is then flexed, externally rotated, and abducted, bringing into view the lesser trochanter. The iliopsoas tendon is exposed, isolated, and divided at its insertion and reflected proximally.

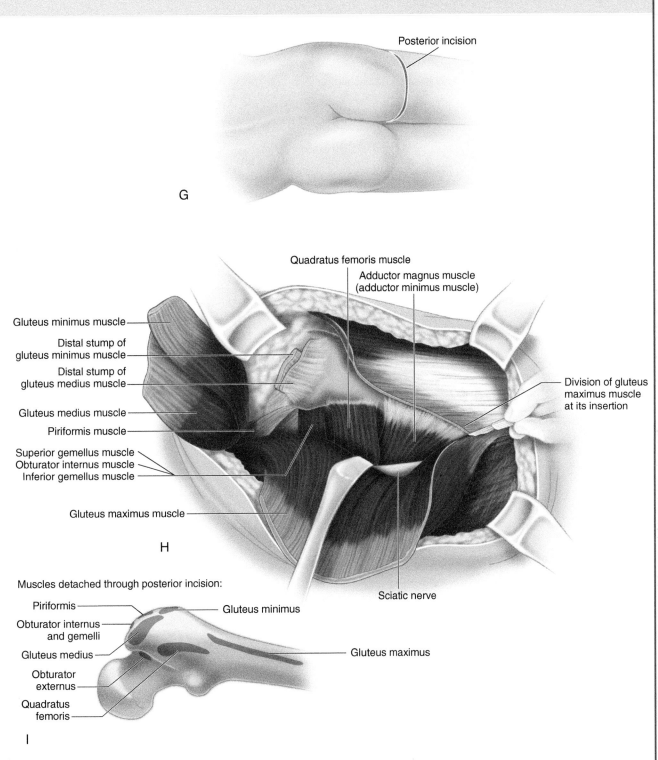

Posterior incision

G

Quadratus femoris muscle

Adductor magnus muscle
(adductor minimus muscle)

Gluteus minimus muscle

Distal stump of
gluteus minimus muscle

Distal stump of
gluteus medius muscle

Gluteus medius muscle

Piriformis muscle

Superior gemellus muscle
Obturator internus muscle
Inferior gemellus muscle

Gluteus maximus muscle

Division of gluteus
maximus muscle
at its insertion

H

Sciatic nerve

Muscles detached through posterior incision:

Piriformis

Gluteus minimus

Obturator internus
and gemelli

Gluteus medius

Gluteus maximus

Obturator
externus

Quadratus
femoris

I

G, To facilitate surgical exposure, a sterile sandbag is placed under the pelvis, and the patient is turned onto the side away from the site of operation. The hip is internally rotated.
H, The gluteus medius and gluteus minimus muscles are divided at their insertion into the greater trochanter and, together with the tensor fasciae latae muscle, reflected proximally. The gluteus maximus muscle is detached at its insertion and retracted upward. The free ends of the gluteus maximus, medius, and minimus muscles and tensor fasciae latae muscle are marked with size 0 silk sutures for reattachment.
I, The muscles to be detached at their insertion through the posterior incision are shown. The short rotators of the hip— that is, the quadratus femoris, obturator externus, gemellus, and obturator internus—are detached from their insertion into the femur.

Continued on following page

Procedure 18   Hip Disarticulation, cont'd

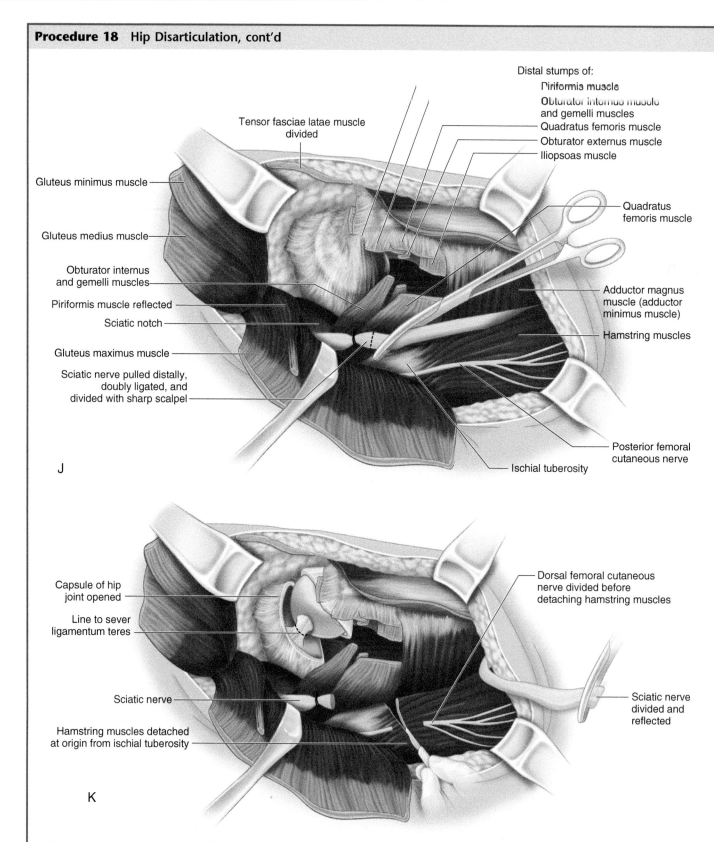

Distal stumps of:
Piriformis muscle
Obturator internus muscle and gemelli muscles
Quadratus femoris muscle
Obturator externus muscle
Iliopsoas muscle

Tensor fasciae latae muscle divided

Gluteus minimus muscle

Gluteus medius muscle

Obturator internus and gemelli muscles

Piriformis muscle reflected

Sciatic notch

Gluteus maximus muscle

Sciatic nerve pulled distally, doubly ligated, and divided with sharp scalpel

Quadratus femoris muscle

Adductor magnus muscle (adductor minimus muscle)

Hamstring muscles

Posterior femoral cutaneous nerve

Ischial tuberosity

J

Capsule of hip joint opened

Line to sever ligamentum teres

Sciatic nerve

Hamstring muscles detached at origin from ischial tuberosity

Dorsal femoral cutaneous nerve divided before detaching hamstring muscles

Sciatic nerve divided and reflected

K

J, The sciatic nerve is identified, dissected free, pulled distally, crushed with a Kocher hemostat at a level 2 inches proximal to the ischial tuberosity, and ligated with size 0 silk sutures to prevent hemorrhage from its accompanying vessels. Next, it is sharply divided just distal to the ligature.

K, The hamstring muscles are detached at their origin from the ischial tuberosity. The capsule of the hip joint is divided near the acetabulum, and the ligamentum teres is severed, completing the disarticulation.

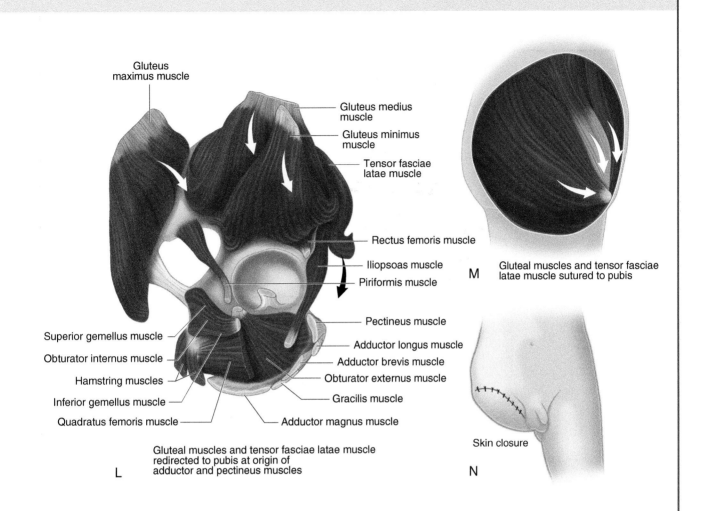

Gluteus maximus muscle

Gluteus medius muscle

Gluteus minimus muscle

Tensor fasciae latae muscle

Rectus femoris muscle

Iliopsoas muscle

Piriformis muscle

Pectineus muscle

Adductor longus muscle

Adductor brevis muscle

Obturator externus muscle

Gracilis muscle

Adductor magnus muscle

Superior gemellus muscle

Obturator internus muscle

Hamstring muscles

Inferior gemellus muscle

Quadratus femoris muscle

Gluteal muscles and tensor fasciae latae muscle redirected to pubis at origin of adductor and pectineus muscles

L

Gluteal muscles and tensor fasciae latae muscle sutured to pubis

M

Skin closure

N

L and **M,** The gluteal flap is mobilized and brought forward, and the free distal ends are sutured to the pubis at the origin of the adductor and pectineus muscles.

N, The wound is closed in routine fashion. A closed suction drain is placed in the inferior portion of the wound. It is removed in 1 to 2 days.

SECTION II

NEUROMUSCULAR DISORDERS

Certain principles and guidelines are helpful in planning surgery in neuromuscular conditions. Children with spastic hemiplegia often walk with a flexed knee and plantar flexed ankle on the affected side. The surgeon can improve their gait significantly by surgically lengthening the medial hamstrings and the tendo-Achilles. On the other hand, a diplegic child with a crouch gait and toe walking may "sink" into further crouch if the heel cords are lengthened. In these children the surgeon should first manage the overactive hip flexors and hamstrings, and carefully lengthen only the gastrocnemius portion of the plantar flexors. Lengthening of the hip flexors should also be approached with caution as these are often the chief motors of gait.

For some years, rectus femoris transfers were frequently done when hamstrings were lengthened to improve knee flexion in swing phase of gait. Fewer transfers are done currently with a concern for quadriceps weakening. The transfer is useful for those with symptomatic lack of knee flexion in gait due to rectus contracture.

Shelf arthroplasties are rarely done for neuromuscular hip dislocation, while more complete procedures including adductor release, varus femoral osteotomy, and acetabular augmentation are used for lasting maintenance of reduction.

In the upper extremity, tendon transfers for cerebral palsy are indicated to improve appearance and function of the extremity. Sensory deficits, especially lack of stereognosis, may often limit functional gains.

Procedure 19   Percutaneous Achilles Tendon Lengthening

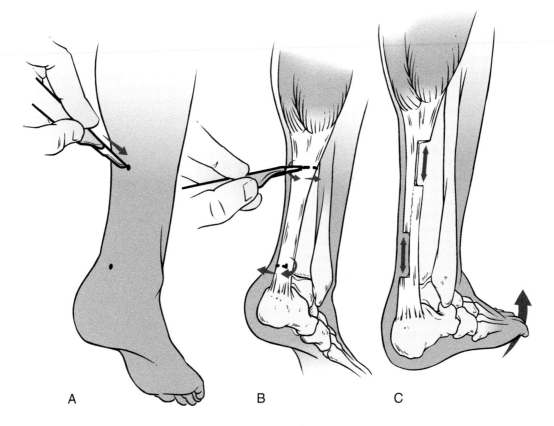

A   B   C

A, The two levels of lengthening are planned. The proximal level should be distal to the musculotendinous junction. The distal level should be close to the insertion into the calcaneus. The distance between the two cuts varies with the severity of the contracture. The knife is inserted through a vertical stab incision into the tendon.

B, The scalpel is then rotated so that slightly more than half the tendon is transected laterally at the proximal site and medially at the distal site.

C, The ankle is then dorsiflexed with gentle pressure until the desired degree of dorsiflexion is obtained. As the tendon lengthens, a "crackling" sound can be heard. If the tendon lengthens suddenly under force, a louder "pop" is heard. The surgeon should squeeze the calf and watch for plantar flexion of the ankle to ensure continuity of the tendon.

D, A short-leg cast and knee immobilizer are then applied.

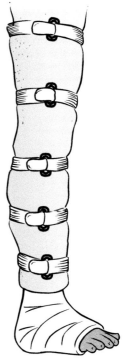

D

Procedure 20   Split Anterior Tibialis Tendon Transfer

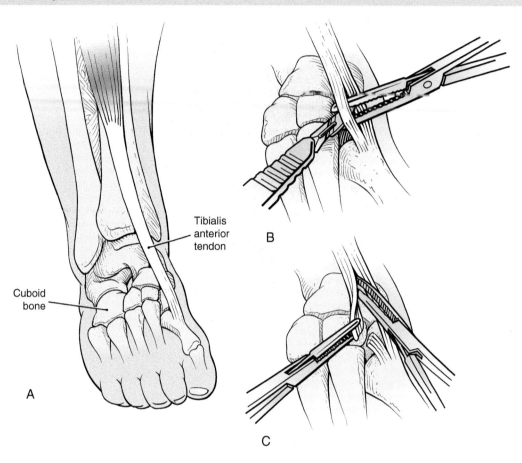

A, A skin incision is made over the insertion of the anterior tibialis at the base of the first metatarsal.

B, A longitudinal split is made in the tendon.
C, The lateral half of the tendon is detached.

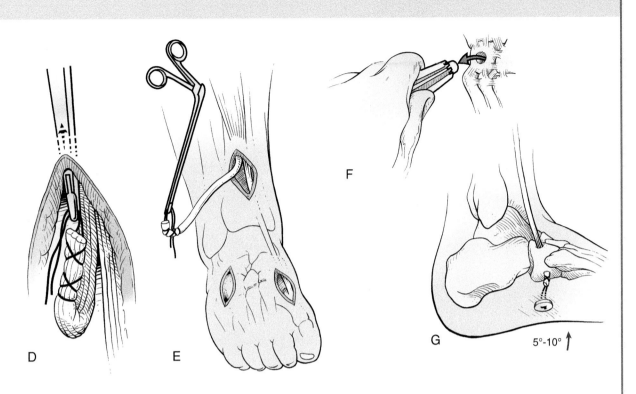

D

E

F

G   5°-10° ↑

D, A stitch is woven into the detached tendon and the split is propagated proximally.

E, A second incision is made over the tibialis anterior just proximal to the extensor retinaculum. With a tendon passer, the split tendon is then delivered on its suture into the proximal wound. A third incision is made over the dorsum of the cuboid.

F, A trephine is used to create a bony tunnel in the cuboid.

G, With the foot held in neutral position, the tendon is transferred into the cuboid and the suture is passed on Keith needles out the sole of the foot. The suture is then tied over felt and a button with tension.

Procedure 21   Extraarticular Arthrodesis of the Subtalar Joint (Grice Procedure)

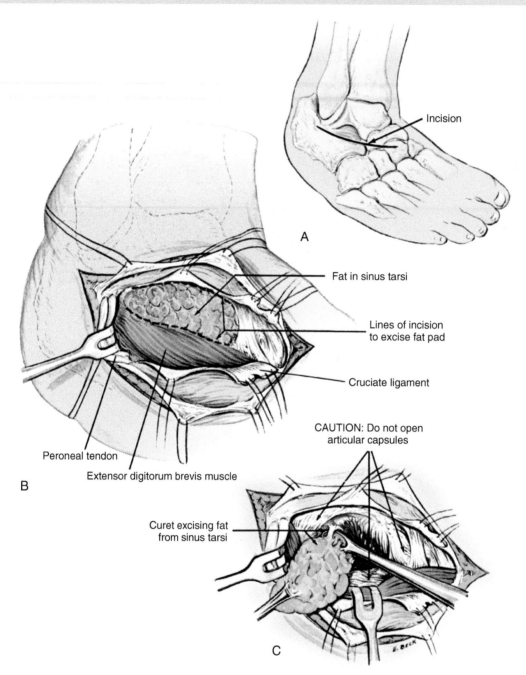

Incision

Fat in sinus tarsi

Lines of incision
to excise fat pad

Cruciate ligament

CAUTION: Do not open
articular capsules

Peroneal tendon

Extensor digitorum brevis muscle

B

Curet excising fat
from sinus tarsi

A

C

A, A 2½-inch-long, slightly curved incision is made over the subtalar joint, centered over the sinus tarsi.
B, The incision is carried down to the sinus tarsi. The capsules of the posterior and anterior subtalar articulations are identified and left intact. The operation is extraarticular. If the capsule is inadvertently opened, it should be closed with interrupted sutures.

The periosteum on the talus corresponding to the lateral margin of the roof of the sinus tarsi is divided and reflected proximally. The fibrofatty tissue in the sinus tarsi and the tendinous origin of the short toe extensors from the calcaneus are elevated and reflected distally in one mass.
C, The remaining fatty and ligamentous tissue from the sinus tarsi is thoroughly removed with a sharp scalpel and curet.

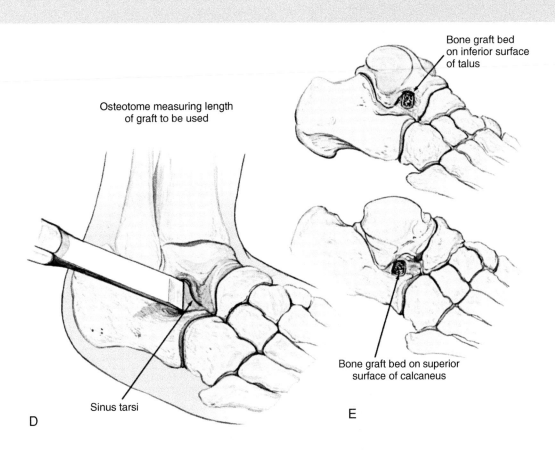

Osteotome measuring length
of graft to be used

Sinus tarsi

D

Bone graft bed
on inferior surface
of talus

Bone graft bed on superior
surface of calcaneus

E

D, Next, the foot is manipulated into equinus position and inversion while rotating the calcaneus into its normal position beneath the talus and correcting the valgus deformity. Broad straight osteotomes of various size ($\frac{3}{4}$ to $1\frac{1}{4}$ inches or more) are inserted into the sinus tarsi to block the subtalar joint and determine the length and optimal position of the bone graft and the stability that it will provide. The long axis of the graft should be parallel to the long axis of the leg when the ankle is dorsiflexed into neutral position.

E, The optimal site of the bone graft bed is marked with a broad osteotome. A thin layer of cortical bone ($\frac{1}{8}$ to $\frac{3}{16}$ inch) is removed with a dental osteotome from the inferior surface of the talus (the roof of the sinus tarsi) and the superior surface of the calcaneus (the floor of the sinus tarsi) at the site marked for the bone graft. It is best to preserve the most lateral cortical margin of the graft bed to support the bone block and prevent it from sinking into soft cancellous bone.

Continued on following page

Procedure 21   Extraarticular Arthrodesis of the Subtalar Joint (Grice Procedure), cont'd

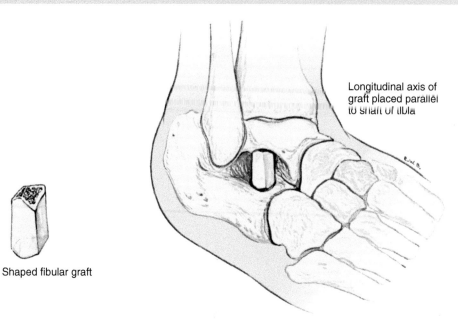

Longitudinal axis of
graft placed parallel
to shaft of tibia

Shaped fibular graft

F

F, A bone graft of appropriate size can be taken from the fibula or iliac crest. The corners of the base of the graft are removed with a rongeur so that the graft is trapezoidal in shape and can be countersunk into cancellous bone to prevent lateral displacement after surgery.

The bone graft is placed in the prepared graft bed in the sinus tarsi by holding the foot in varus position. An impactor may be used to fix the cortices of the graft in place. The longitudinal axis of the graft should be parallel to the shaft of the tibia with the ankle in neutral position.

With the foot held in the desired position, the distal soft tissue pedicle of fibrofatty tissue of the sinus tarsi, the calcaneal periosteum, and the tendinous origin of the short toe extensors are sutured to the reflected periosteum from the talus. The subcutaneous tissue and skin are closed with interrupted sutures, and a below-knee cast is applied.

Postoperative Care

The cast is removed 8 to 10 weeks after surgery. If radiographs show solid healing of the graft, gradual weight bearing is allowed with the protection of crutches. Active and passive exercises are performed to strengthen the muscles and increase range of motion of the ankle and knee.

Procedure 22 **Lateral Column Lengthening**

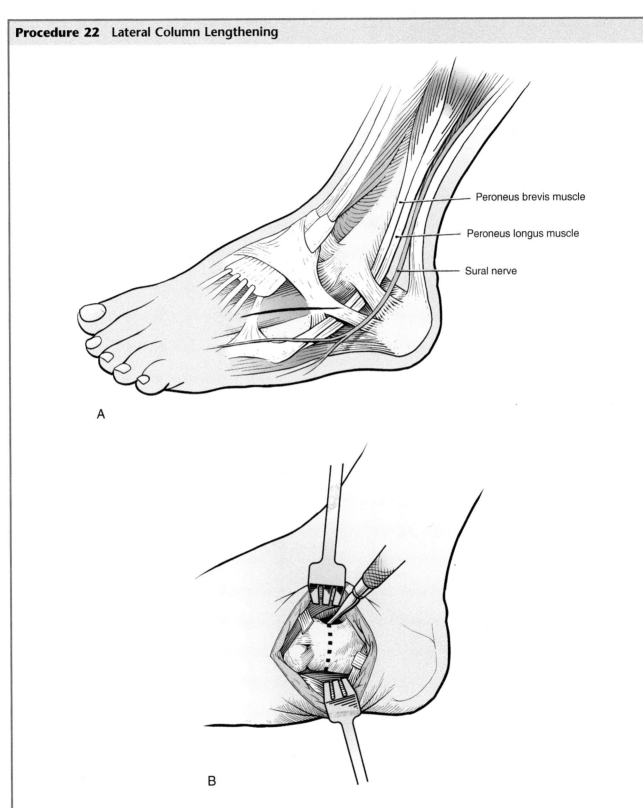

A

A, The calcaneus is approached laterally through a longitudinal incision.

B

B, The peroneal tendons are retracted plantarward and the neck of the calcaneus is exposed. The calcaneocuboid joint is identified but left undisturbed.

Continued on following page

Procedure 22 Lateral Column Lengthening, cont'd

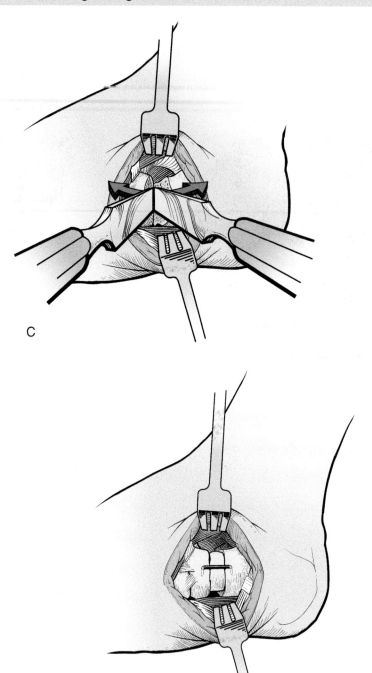

C

D

C, A vertical osteotomy is made in the neck of the calcaneus and hinged open laterally with osteotomes. A lamina spreader should not be used because it will crush the bony fragments.

D, A tricortical wedge of iliac crest is placed in the osteotomy. The osteotomy may be stabilized with K-wires or a staple.

Procedure 23   Hamstring Lengthening

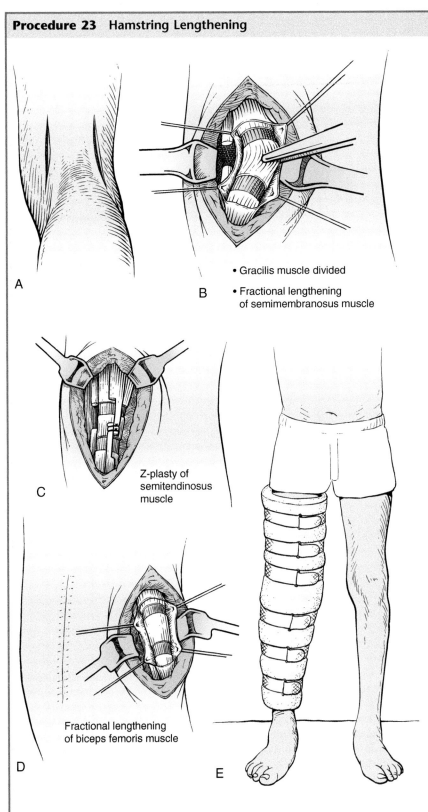

- Gracilis muscle divided

- Fractional lengthening of semimembranosus muscle

Z-plasty of semitendinosus muscle

Fractional lengthening of biceps femoris muscle

A, The hamstrings are approached through two longitudinal incisions. The medial incision is placed over the gracilis tendon and the lateral incision is placed lateral to the biceps femoris to protect the peroneal nerve.

B, All three medial hamstrings are first identified. After this step the gracilis tendon may be divided or lengthened. The aponeurosis of the semimembranosus is cut while the underlying muscle fibers are left in continuity. Usually, two cuts in the aponeurosis spaced approximately 1.5 to 2.0 cm apart are required. By gently extending the patient's knee and flexing the hip, the surgeon can perform a sliding lengthening.

C, The semitendinosus tendon is lengthened with a Z-plasty and repaired.

D, The biceps femoris is identified and the peroneal nerve protected because it lies directly medial and deep to the tendon. An intramuscular lengthening procedure is performed by incising just the tendinous portion of the biceps while leaving the muscular fibers in continuity, as was done for the semimembranosus lengthening. Again, the hip is flexed and the knee extended to achieve a sliding lengthening.

E, The patient is then placed either in a knee immobilizer or in a long-leg cast with a straight knee. When other tendon or bone surgery is performed simultaneously, the mode of immobilization may vary. Early mobilization and weight bearing are encouraged.

Procedure 24 (Video 6)   Rectus Femoris Transfer

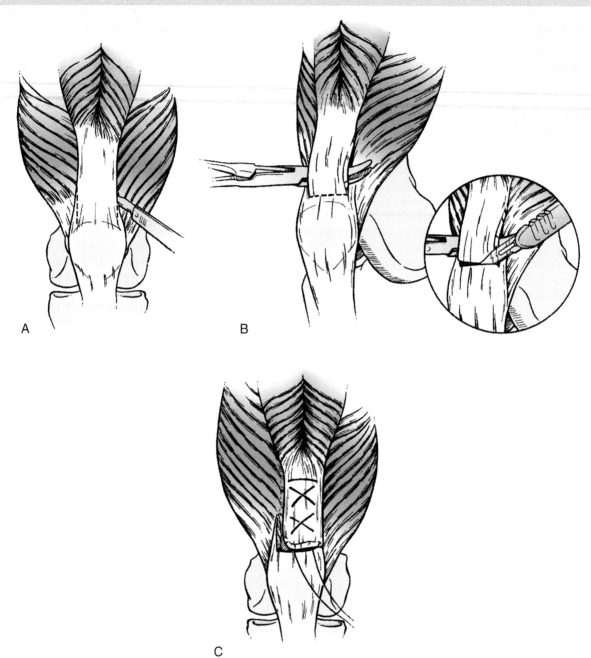

A

B

C

A, The incision may be either a horizontal incision two fingerbreadths proximal to the proximal pole of the patella or a vertical incision. The conjoined quadriceps tendon is isolated and the rectus femoris component is identified. The rectus tendon is separated from the tendinous portions of the vastus medialis and lateralis.

B, The undersurface of the rectus must be carefully separated from the intermedius. This step is most easily done proximally and extended by following the plane to the insertion on the patella. The rectus tendon can then be sharply released from the patella.
C, A strong suture is woven into the rectus tendon to be used in the transfer.

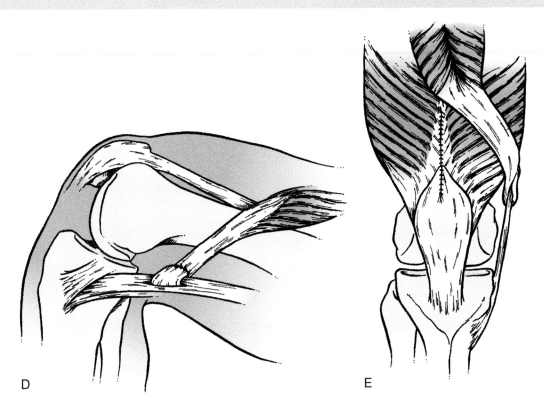

D

E

D, A medial posterior longitudinal incision is made and the gracilis tendon is isolated. The rectus is mobilized and transferred back into the posterior wound by grasping the suture. The tendon is then routed subcutaneously. The distal end of the rectus tendon is inserted through the tendon selected for the site of transfer and sutured back onto itself. The gracilis is a popular site for the transfer, but use of the sartorius and biceps femoris has also been described.

E, The vastus medialis and lateralis may be repaired to each other to re-create the quadriceps tendon. The patient can be immobilized either in a long-leg cast or in a knee immobilizer.

Procedure 25   Adductor Contracture Release

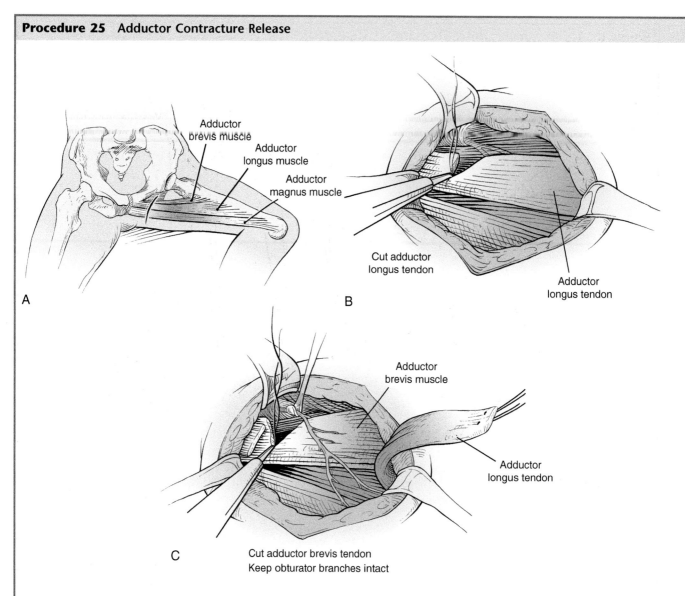

A — Adductor brevis muscle / Adductor longus muscle / Adductor magnus muscle

B — Cut adductor longus tendon / Adductor longus tendon

C — Adductor brevis muscle / Adductor longus tendon / Cut adductor brevis tendon / Keep obturator branches intact

A, A transverse incision is made in the groin crease and centered over the adductor longus tendon, which is easily palpated.
B, The adductor longus tendon is identified, isolated from the deeper adductor brevis, and divided with electrocautery.

C, The adductor brevis is then divided in part with electrocautery. Care is taken to identify the anterior branch of the obturator nerve, which should be preserved. The posterior branch of the obturator nerve, which lies deep to the adductor brevis, should likewise be preserved.

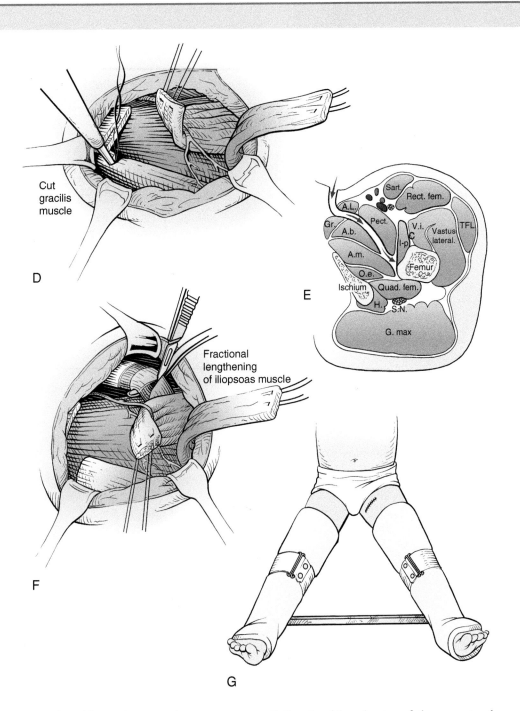

D, Just posterior to the adductor brevis and more superficial, the gracilis is identified. This flat, broad muscle is released from its origin with electrocautery.

E, If concomitant release of the iliopsoas is performed in a nonambulatory child, its tendinous insertion on the lesser trochanter can be palpated deep to the adductor brevis.

F, Fractional lengthening of the psoas tendon can be performed at this level, as illustrated, or preferably more proximally at the pelvic brim.

G, Immobilization consists of two long-leg casts with a removable abduction bar. The bar can be removed for range-of-motion exercises and transport but should be used most of the day for 3 to 4 weeks. The hip flexion contracture release is best treated by placing the child in the prone position at frequent intervals.

Procedure 26   **Shelf Acetabular Augmentation**

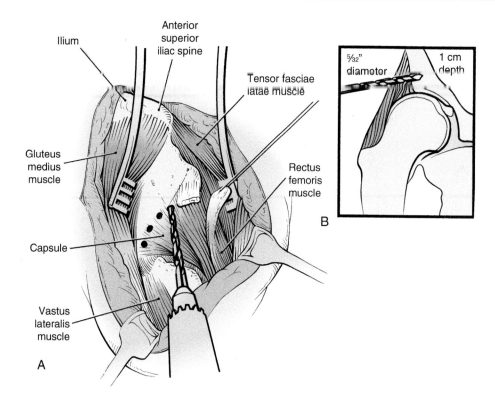

A, The patient is positioned supine with a bump beneath the affected hip. Through an anterior approach, the outer table of the ilium is exposed down to the hip capsule. The rectus femoris is detached and tagged. After verifying the position with fluoroscopy, the surgeon uses a drill to outline the shelf just superior to the acetabular rim along the lateral aspect of the hip.

B, The drill is inserted approximately 1 cm just above the capsule.

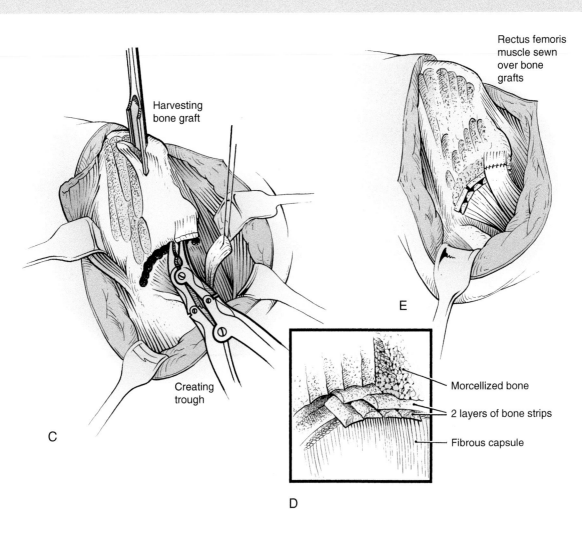

Harvesting
bone graft

Creating
trough

C

Rectus femoris
muscle sewn
over bone
grafts

E

Morcellized bone

2 layers of bone strips

Fibrous capsule

D

C, A rongeur is used to connect the holes to create a trough for bone graft. Strips of corticocancellous and cancellous graft are obtained from the iliac wing. The graft is placed in the trough and over the hip capsule to form an awning covering the femoral head.

D, The strips are placed at 90-degree angles in layers, and morcellized bone graft is extended up the iliac wing.
E, The rectus femoris is repaired over the shelf and a spica cast applied.

Procedure 27 **Dega Osteotomy**

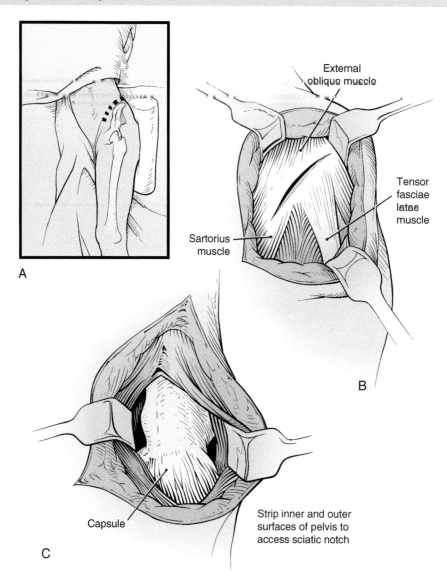

A

External oblique muscle

Tensor fasciae latae muscle

Sartorius muscle

B

Capsule

Strip inner and outer surfaces of pelvis to access sciatic notch

C

A, The patient is positioned supine with the affected hip raised on a bump. An anterior incision is made over the iliac crest. The Dega osteotomy is usually performed during the same surgical setting as a varus derotation osteotomy and will be illustrated as such.

B and **C,** The iliac apophysis is split and the inner and outer tables are exposed subperiosteally to the sciatic notch. The direct head of the rectus femoris is detached.

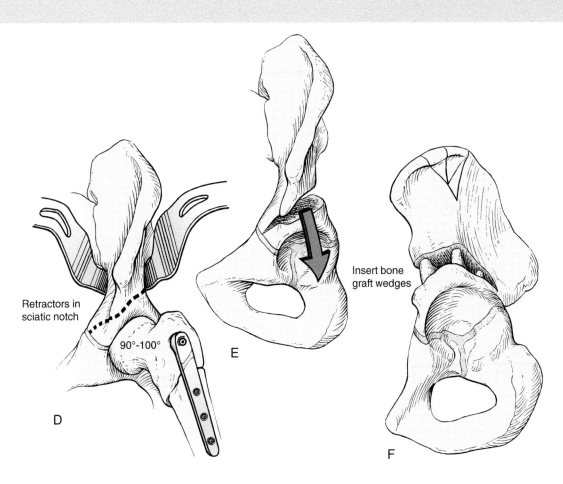

D, Blunt Hohmann retractors are placed in the sciatic notch. The osteotomy is drawn on the pelvis at the level of the anterior inferior iliac spine and extended back to the sciatic notch.

E, Osteotomes are then inserted from the outer table of the ilium down to the triradiate cartilage. The inner table is preserved. The anterior inferior iliac spine is cut with the osteotome, and the sciatic notch is incised with a Kerrison rongeur. The acetabulum is pried inferiorly and laterally with osteotomes. If a lamina spreader is used, great care should be taken so that the bony surfaces are not crushed.

F, Tricortical wedges of iliac crest are harvested and stacked in the opening wedge of the osteotomy. The graft can be preferentially positioned to improve coverage more anteriorly, posteriorly, or just laterally. If the inner table remains intact, the osteotomy does not require fixation. Ranging the hip under visualization is recommended to verify that the osteotomy is stable. A spica cast is then used for 6 weeks to allow healing of the osteotomy.

Procedure 28   Anterior Transfer of the Posterior Tibial Tendon Through the Interosseous Membrane

Operative Technique

A, A 4-cm-long incision is made over the medial aspect of the foot, beginning posterior and immediately distal to the tip of the medial malleolus and extending to the base of the first cuneiform bone. A second longitudinal incision is made 1.5 cm posterior to the subcutaneous medial border of the tibia and ends 3 cm from the tip of the medial malleolus.

B, The posterior tibial tendon is identified at its insertion, and its sheath is divided. The tendon is freed and sectioned at its attachment to the bone, with maximal length preserved. A 0-0 silk whip suture is inserted in its distal end.

C, The posterior tibial muscle is identified through the leg incision, and its sheath is opened and freed. Traction on the stump in the foot incision can help in its identification. Moist sponges and a two-hand technique are used to deliver the posterior tibial tendon into the proximal wound. The surgeon must be careful to preserve the nerve and blood supply to the posterior tibial muscle.

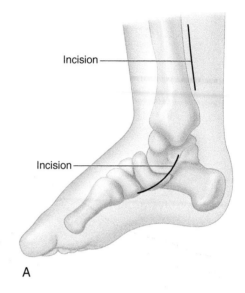

A

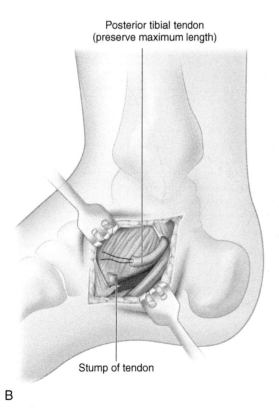

Posterior tibial tendon
(preserve maximum length)

Stump of tendon

B

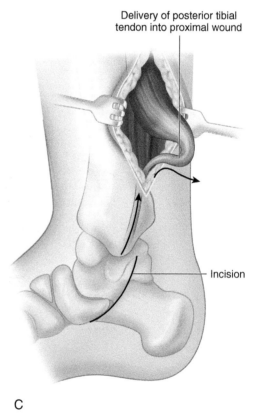

Delivery of posterior tibial
tendon into proximal wound

Incision

C

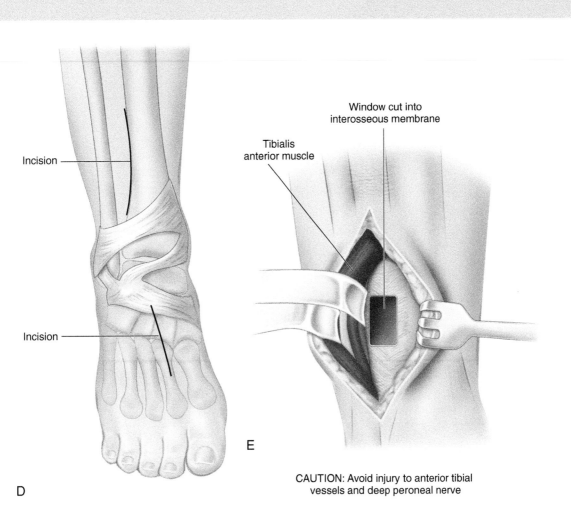

D, A longitudinal skin incision is made anteriorly one fingerbreadth lateral to the crest of the tibia, starting at the proximal margin of the cruciate ligament of the ankle and extending 7 cm proximally. A 4-cm-long longitudinal incision is then made over the dorsum of the foot, centered over the base of the second metatarsal.

E, The anterior tibial muscle is exposed together with the anterior tibial artery and extensor hallucis longus muscle. It is retracted laterally to expose the interosseous membrane. Next, a large rectangular window is cut in the interosseous membrane.

Continued on following page

Procedure 28   Anterior Transfer of the Posterior Tibial Tendon Through the Interosseous Membrane, cont'd

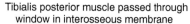

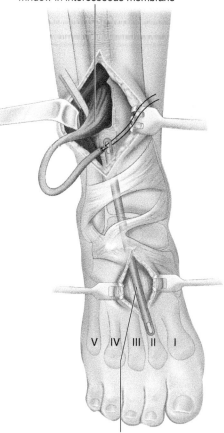

Tibialis posterior muscle passed through window in interosseous membrane

V IV III II I

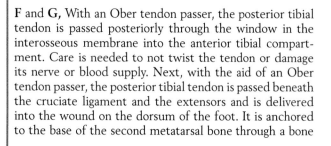

Ober tendon passer delivers tibialis posterior tendon beneath extensors and cruciate ligament into wound over base of second metatarsal

F

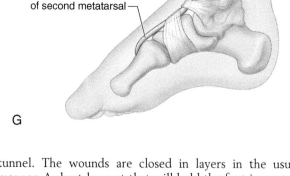

Tibialis posterior tendon anchored into base of second metatarsal

G

F and G, With an Ober tendon passer, the posterior tibial tendon is passed posteriorly through the window in the interosseous membrane into the anterior tibial compartment. Care is needed to not twist the tendon or damage its nerve or blood supply. Next, with the aid of an Ober tendon passer, the posterior tibial tendon is passed beneath the cruciate ligament and the extensors and is delivered into the wound on the dorsum of the foot. It is anchored to the base of the second metatarsal bone through a bone

tunnel. The wounds are closed in layers in the usual manner. A short-leg cast that will hold the foot in neutral position at the ankle joint is applied.

Postoperative Care

The principles of postoperative care are the same as for any tendon transfer.

Procedure 29   Achilles Tendon—Distal Fibular Tenodesis for Mild Ankle Valgus in Skeletally Immature Patients

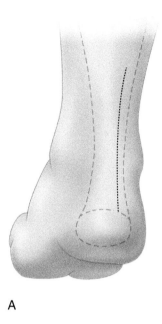

A

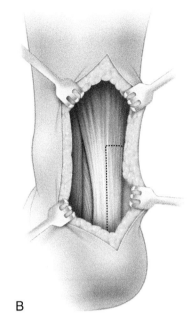

B

The patient is placed prone on the operating table for easiest exposure of the posterior aspect of the lower leg and heel.

Operative Technique

A, A long vertical incision is made, paralleling the lateral border of the Achilles tendon. Through this incision, the Achilles tendon, peroneal tendons, and posterior aspect of the fibular shaft proximal to its physis are exposed.

B, A distally based slip (≈1 cm wide) of Achilles tendon is fashioned. The remaining Achilles tendon is lengthened if necessary.

Continued on following page

Procedure 29   Achilles Tendon—Distal Fibular Tenodesis for Mild Ankle Valgus in Skeletally Immature Patients, cont'd

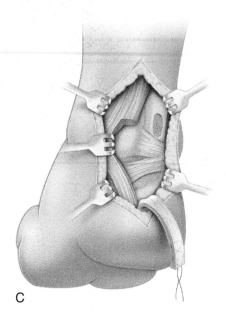
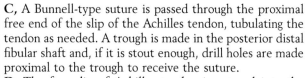

C

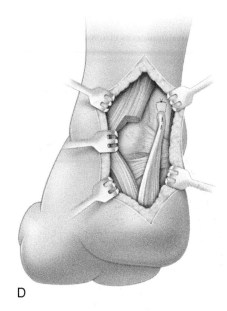

D

C, A Bunnell-type suture is passed through the proximal free end of the slip of the Achilles tendon, tubulating the tendon as needed. A trough is made in the posterior distal fibular shaft and, if it is stout enough, drill holes are made proximal to the trough to receive the suture.

D, The free slip of Achilles tendon is sutured into the trough in the distal fibula. The transferred portion of the Achilles tendon should be tensioned so that it is snug in neutral ankle dorsiflexion. If the fibula is too small for holes to be drilled in the cortex, the suture can be passed around the shaft of the fibula or the slip of Achilles tendon can be wrapped around the fibula and sutured to itself. The wounds are irrigated and closed. A well-molded and padded short-leg walking cast is applied with the foot in a neutral position.

Postoperative Management

The patient is allowed to bear weight in the cast. The child and parents are educated to watch for evidence of skin irritation or excoriation at the edges of the cast and tips of the toes and to report breakdown of the sole of the cast. The cast is removed 6 weeks after surgery, and the patient is placed in ankle-foot or knee-ankle-foot orthoses, as needed.

Procedure 30   Iliopsoas Muscle Transfer for Paralysis of the Hip Abductors

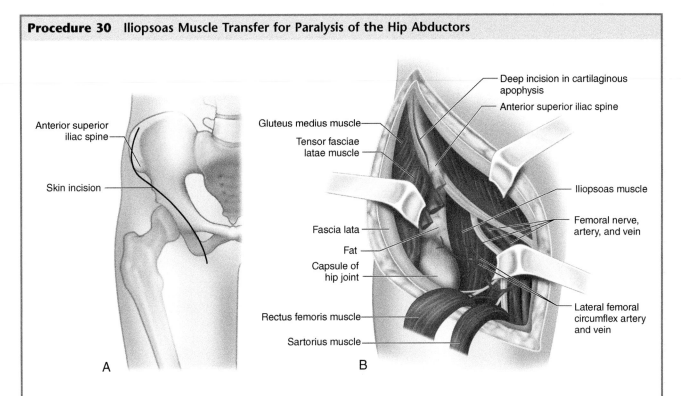

Operative Technique

The patient is positioned supine with a small sandbag under the sacrum and a larger sandbag under the ipsilateral scapula. The entire involved lower limb, the hip, the lower part of the abdomen and chest, and the iliac and sacral regions are prepared in sterile fashion and draped so that the limb that is to be operated on can be freely manipulated and the incision extended to the posterior third of the iliac crest without contamination.

A, The skin incision extends forward from the junction of the posterior and middle thirds of the iliac crest to the anterior superior iliac spine; it is then carried distally into the thigh along the medial border of the sartorius muscle for a distance of 10 to 12 cm and ends 2 cm distal to the lesser trochanter.

B, The deep fascia is incised over the iliac crest, and the fascia lata is opened in line with the skin incision.

The lateral femoral cutaneous nerve is identified; it usually crosses the sartorius muscle 2.5 cm distal to the anterior superior iliac spine and lies in close proximity to the lateral border of the sartorius. The nerve is mobilized by sharp dissection and protected by retracting it medially with moist hernia tape. The wound flaps are undermined and retracted. The anterior medial margin of the tensor fasciae latae muscle is identified, and by blunt dissection, the groove between the sartorius and rectus femoris muscles medially and the tensor fasciae latae muscle laterally is opened. The dissection is carried deep through the loose areolar tissue that separates these structures, and the adipose tissue that covers the front of the capsule of the hip joint is exposed. The ascending branch of the lateral femoral circumflex artery and the accompanying vein cross the midportion of the wound; they are isolated, clamped, cut, and ligated.

The origin of the sartorius muscle from the anterior superior iliac spine is detached and the muscle is reflected distally and medially. The free end is marked with a silk whip suture for later reattachment. The origins of the two heads of the rectus femoris are divided and reflected distally. The femoral nerve and its branches to the sartorius and rectus femoris are identified. Moist hernia tape is passed around the femoral nerve for gentle handling. The femoral vessels and nerve are retracted medially.

Continued on following page

Procedure 30   Iliopsoas Muscle Transfer for Paralysis of the Hip Abductors, cont'd

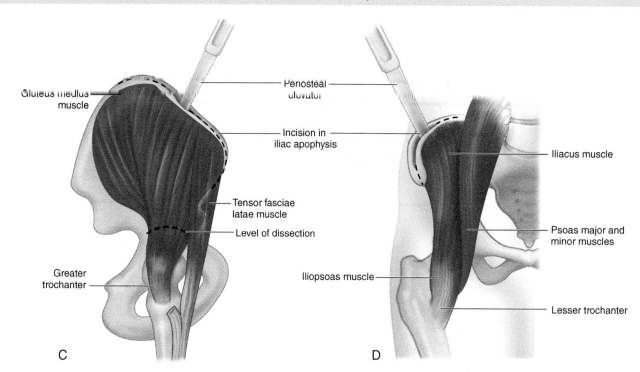

C

D

C, The cartilaginous apophysis of the ilium is split and the dissection is deepened along the iliac crest down to bone. With a broad periosteal elevator the tensor fasciae latae and the gluteus medius and minimus muscles are stripped subperiosteally from the lateral surface of the ilium and reflected in one continuous mass laterally and distally to the superior margin of the acetabulum. Bleeding is controlled by packing the interval between the reflected muscles and ilium with laparotomy pads.

D, Then, with a large periosteal elevator, the iliacus muscle is subperiosteally elevated and reflected medially to expose the inner wall of the wing of the ilium from the greater sciatic notch to the anterior superior iliac spine.

By careful blunt dissection with a periosteal elevator, the iliacus muscle is freed, elevated, and mobilized from the inner wall of the ilium and the anterior capsule of the hip joint. It is important to stay lateral and deep to the iliacus muscle and work in a proximal-to-distal direction.

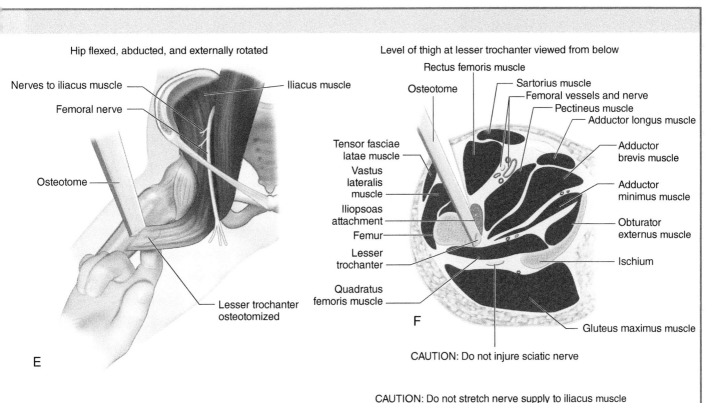

Hip flexed, abducted, and externally rotated

Nerves to iliacus muscle

Femoral nerve

Iliacus muscle

Osteotome

Lesser trochanter osteotomized

E

Level of thigh at lesser trochanter viewed from below

Rectus femoris muscle

Osteotome

Sartorius muscle

Femoral vessels and nerve

Pectineus muscle

Adductor longus muscle

Tensor fasciae latae muscle

Vastus lateralis muscle

Iliopsoas attachment

Femur

Lesser trochanter

Quadratus femoris muscle

Adductor brevis muscle

Adductor minimus muscle

Obturator externus muscle

Ischium

Gluteus maximus muscle

F

CAUTION: Do not injure sciatic nerve

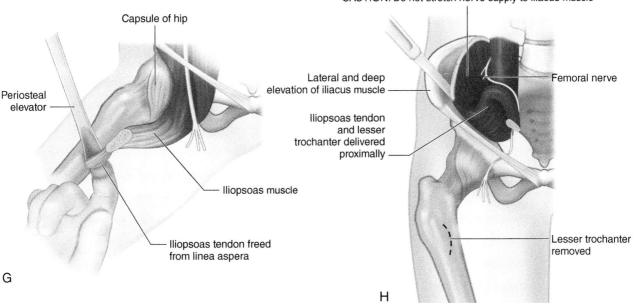

Capsule of hip

Periosteal elevator

Iliopsoas muscle

Iliopsoas tendon freed from linea aspera

G

CAUTION: Do not stretch nerve supply to iliacus muscle

Lateral and deep elevation of iliacus muscle

Iliopsoas tendon and lesser trochanter delivered proximally

Femoral nerve

Lesser trochanter removed

H

E to G, Next the hip is flexed, abducted, and laterally rotated, and with the index finger the lesser trochanter is cleared of soft tissues proximally, posteriorly, and distally. The index finger is then placed on the posteromedial aspect of the lesser trochanter and is used to direct a curved osteotome to the superior and deep aspect of the base of the lesser trochanter.

The lesser trochanter is osteotomized and the distal insertion of the iliacus muscle on the linea aspera of the femur is freed with a periosteal elevator.

H, The iliacus and psoas muscles are reflected proximally by sharp and dull dissection. It is essential to avoid injuring the nerve to the iliacus, which at times enters the muscle belly distally; in addition, the femoral nerve should not be damaged. We find the use of a nerve stimulator of great help. Circumflex vessels are clamped, cut, and ligated as necessary.

Continued on following page

Procedure 30   Iliopsoas Muscle Transfer for Paralysis of the Hip Abductors, cont'd

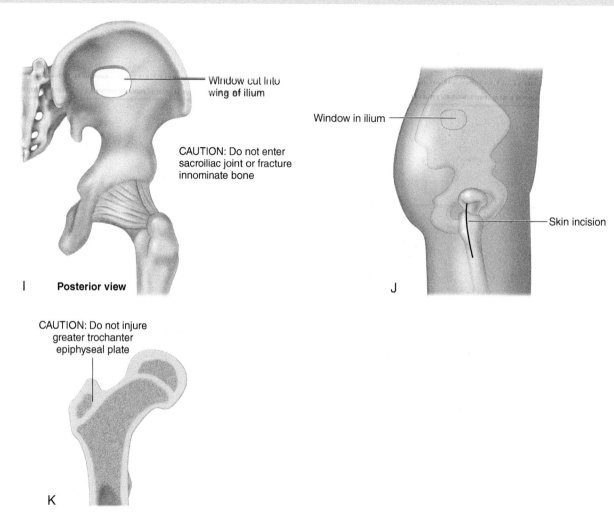

I, Posterior view

Window cut into wing of ilium

CAUTION: Do not enter sacroiliac joint or fracture innominate bone

Window in ilium

Skin incision

J

CAUTION: Do not injure greater trochanter epiphyseal plate

K

I, In the middle third of the wing of the ilium a rectangular hole, usually 1 to 2 in, is cut with drill holes and osteotomes. The hole should be large enough to accommodate the transferred muscle. It should be located as far posteriorly as possible to allow a more direct line of muscle action. The limiting factor is the nerve supply to the iliacus, which should not be stretched.

J, With the hip in extension and medial rotation, the greater trochanter is exposed via a longitudinal lateral incision. The vastus lateralis muscle is split and the lateral surface of the proximal 4 to 5 cm of femoral shaft is subperiosteally exposed.

K, It is important to avoid damaging the apophyseal growth plate of the greater trochanter.

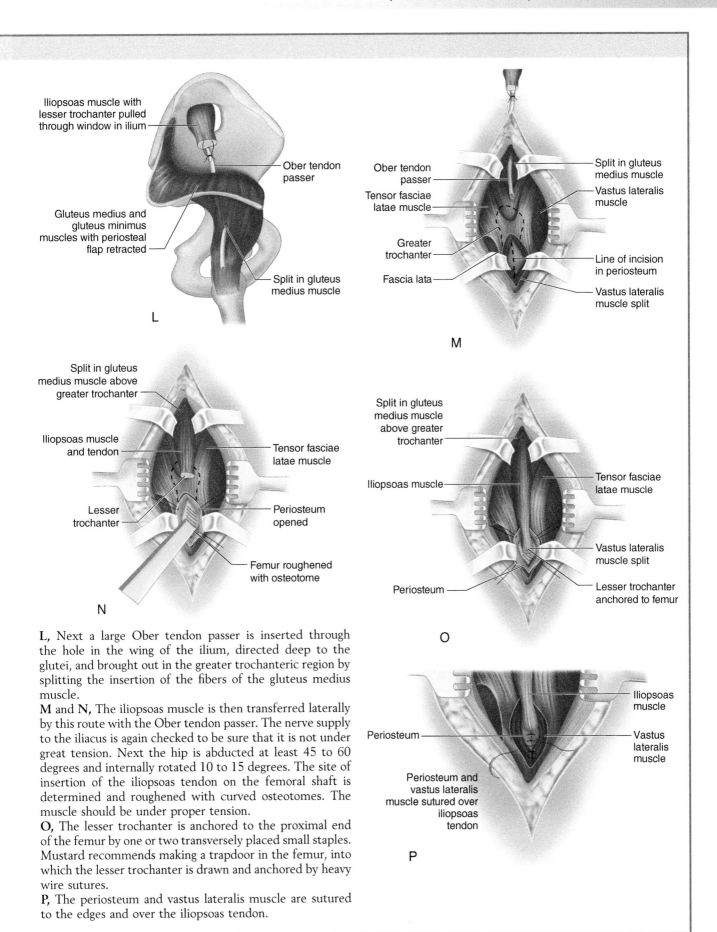

L, Next a large Ober tendon passer is inserted through the hole in the wing of the ilium, directed deep to the glutei, and brought out in the greater trochanteric region by splitting the insertion of the fibers of the gluteus medius muscle.

M and N, The iliopsoas muscle is then transferred laterally by this route with the Ober tendon passer. The nerve supply to the iliacus is again checked to be sure that it is not under great tension. Next the hip is abducted at least 45 to 60 degrees and internally rotated 10 to 15 degrees. The site of insertion of the iliopsoas tendon on the femoral shaft is determined and roughened with curved osteotomes. The muscle should be under proper tension.

O, The lesser trochanter is anchored to the proximal end of the femur by one or two transversely placed small staples. Mustard recommends making a trapdoor in the femur, into which the lesser trochanter is drawn and anchored by heavy wire sutures.

P, The periosteum and vastus lateralis muscle are sutured to the edges and over the iliopsoas tendon.

Continued on following page

Procedure 30   Iliopsoas Muscle Transfer for Paralysis of the Hip Abductors, cont'd

Reattachment of muscles

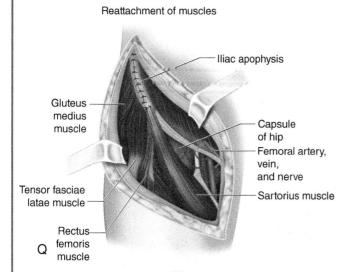

Iliac apophysis

Gluteus medius muscle

Capsule of hip

Femoral artery, vein, and nerve

Tensor fasciae latae muscle

Sartorius muscle

Rectus femoris muscle

Q

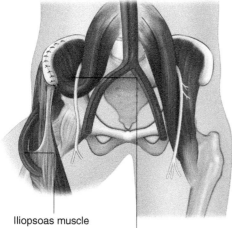

Iliopsoas muscle

R

Iliopsoas muscle pulled through window in ilium

Q and **R,** The rectus femoris and sartorius muscles are sutured to the inferior and superior iliac spines, respectively. The tensor fasciae latae, gluteus medius and minimus, and abdominal muscles are sutured to the iliac crest. The wound is closed in layers in routine manner. A one-and-one-half hip spica cast is applied with the hip in 60 degrees of abduction, 10 to 15 degrees of medial rotation, and slight flexion.

Postoperative Care

Four to 6 weeks after surgery, the patient is readmitted to the hospital, the cast is removed, and a new bivalved hip spica cast is made. It should be cut low on the lateral side so that hip abduction exercises can be performed in the posterior half of the cast. Radiographs of the hips are obtained to determine the stability of the hip joint. Great care should be exercised to avoid causing a pathologic fracture of the femur when the child is lifted out of the cast.

Training of the iliopsoas transfer follows the same general principles as training of tendon transfers in poliomyelitis. In myelomeningocele, however, extensive paralysis of the lower limb necessitates orthotic support, and the patient is much younger. Thus as soon as the transferred iliopsoas has fair motor strength and the lower limbs can be adducted to neutral position, weight bearing is permitted in bilateral above-knee orthoses. The butterfly pelvic band keeps the hips in 5 to 10 degrees of abduction during locomotion. At night, the hips and the transfer are protected in the bivalved hip spica cast or in a plastic hip-knee-ankle-foot orthosis.

Procedure 31   **Anterior Transfer of the Peroneus Longus Tendon to the Base of the Second Metatarsal**

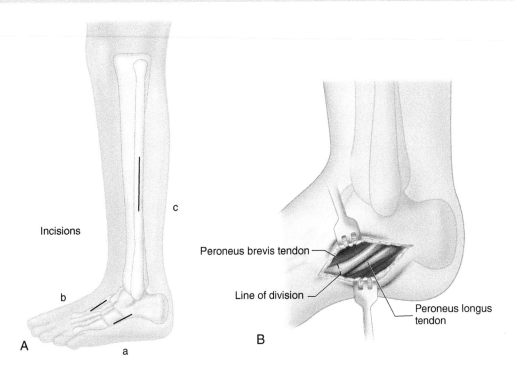

Operative Technique

The patient is placed in a semilateral position with a sandbag under the hip on the affected side.

A, A 3- to 4-cm-long incision (*a*) is made over the lateral aspect of the foot from the base of the fifth metatarsal to a point 1 cm distal to the tip of the lateral malleolus. Subcutaneous tissue is divided, and the tendons of the peroneus longus and brevis are exposed. A second incision (*c*) is then made over the fibular aspect of the leg; it begins 3 cm above the lateral malleolus and extends proximally for a distance of 7 cm. Subcutaneous tissue and deep fascia are incised, and the peroneal tendons are exposed by dividing their sheath. The peroneus longus tendon lies superficial to that of the peroneus brevis. The muscle is inspected to ensure that it is of normal gross appearance.

B, Next the peroneus brevis muscle is detached from the base of the fifth metatarsal and a whip suture is inserted into its distal end.

Continued on following page

Procedure 31   Anterior Transfer of the Peroneus Longus Tendon to the Base of the Second Metatarsal, cont'd

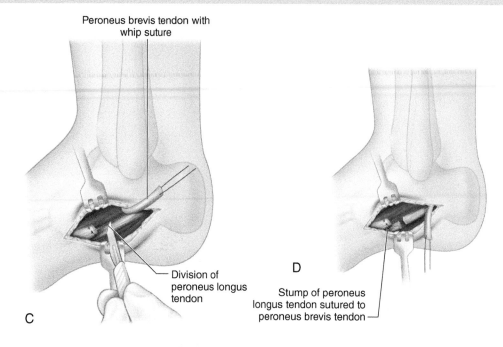

Peroneus brevis tendon with whip suture

Division of peroneus longus tendon

C

D

Stump of peroneus longus tendon sutured to peroneus brevis tendon

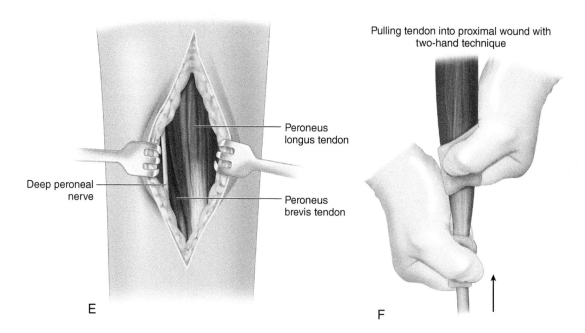

Deep peroneal nerve

Peroneus longus tendon

Peroneus brevis tendon

E

Pulling tendon into proximal wound with two-hand technique

F

C and **D,** The peroneus longus tendon is divided as far distally as possible. The peroneus brevis tendon is sutured to the distal stump of the peroneus longus tendon to preserve the longitudinal arch and depression of the first metatarsal.

E and **F,** The peroneus longus tendon is mobilized and, with a two-hand technique, gently pulled into the proximal wound in the leg. The origin of the peroneus brevis tendon from the fibula should not be disrupted. An adequate opening is made in the intermuscular septum with care taken not to injure any neurovascular structures.

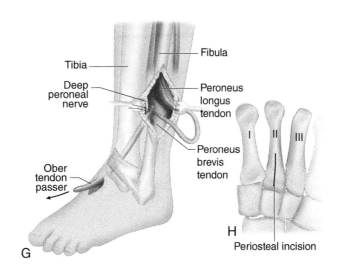

Technique of anchoring tendon to bone

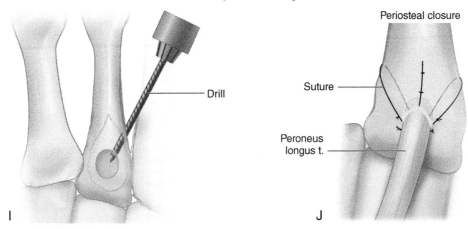

G and **H,** A 2- to 3-cm-long longitudinal incision is made over the dorsum of the foot (incision *b* in part **A**), centered over the base of the second metatarsal. The deep fascia is divided, and the extensor tendons are retracted to expose the proximal fourth of the second metatarsal. The periosteum is divided longitudinally and the cortex of the recipient bone is exposed.

With an Ober tendon passer, the peroneus longus tendon along with its sheath is passed into the anterior tibial compartment, deep to the cruciate crural and tarsal ligaments, and delivered into the incision on the dorsum of the foot. We do not recommend a subcutaneous route. A direct line of pull of the peroneus longus tendon from its origin to its insertion should be ensured.

I and **J,** A drill hole is made in the base of the second metatarsal. A star-head hand drill is used to enlarge the hole to receive the tendon adequately. The peroneus longus tendon is passed through the recipient hole and sutured on itself under correct tension. If the peroneus longus tendon is not of adequate length, two small holes are made 1.5 cm distal to the large hole at each side of the metatarsal shaft. The silk sutures at the end of the tendon are passed from the large central hole to the lateral distal small holes and the tendon is securely sutured to the bone. The ankle joint should be in neutral position or 5 degrees of dorsiflexion. The pneumatic tourniquet is released and hemostasis is obtained. The wounds are closed in routine manner. A long-leg cast is applied with the ankle in 5 degrees of dorsiflexion and the knee in 45 degrees of flexion. Postoperative care follows the guidelines outlined in the section on the principles of tendon transfer.

Procedure 32   **Posterior Tendon Transfer to the Os Calcis for Correction of Calcaneus Deformity (Green and Grice Procedure)**

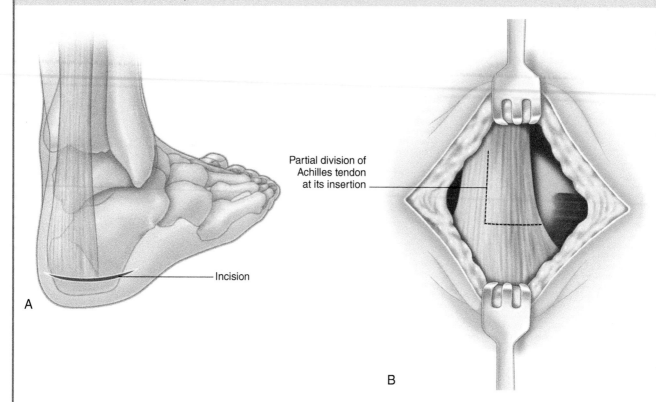

Partial division of Achilles tendon at its insertion

Incision

A

B

Operative Technique

It is best to place the patient in the prone position to facilitate surgical exposure of the heel. The posterior tibial and peroneus longus and brevis tendons are divided distally at their insertion and delivered into the proximal wound. When the flexor hallucis longus tendon is to be transferred, its distal portion is sutured to the flexor hallucis brevis muscle. The anterior tibial tendon is delivered into the calf and heel through the interosseous route.

A, A 5-cm-long posterior transverse incision is made around the heel along one of the skin creases in the part that neither presses the shoe nor touches the ground.

B, The skin and subcutaneous flaps are undercut and reflected to expose the os calcis and the insertion of the Achilles tendon. An L-shaped cut is made in the lateral two thirds of the insertion of the Achilles tendon. The divided portion is reflected proximally to expose the apophysis of the os calcis.

C, Next, with a ⁹⁄₆₄-in drill, a hole is made through the calcaneus, beginning in the center of the apophysis and coming out laterally at its plantar aspect. With a diamond-head hand drill and curet, the hole is enlarged to receive all the transferred tendons.

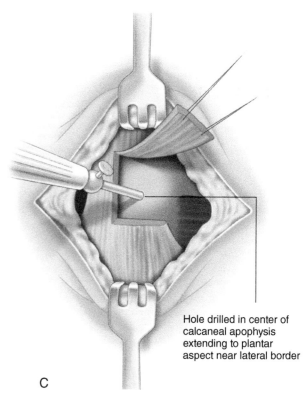

Hole drilled in center of calcaneal apophysis extending to plantar aspect near lateral border

C

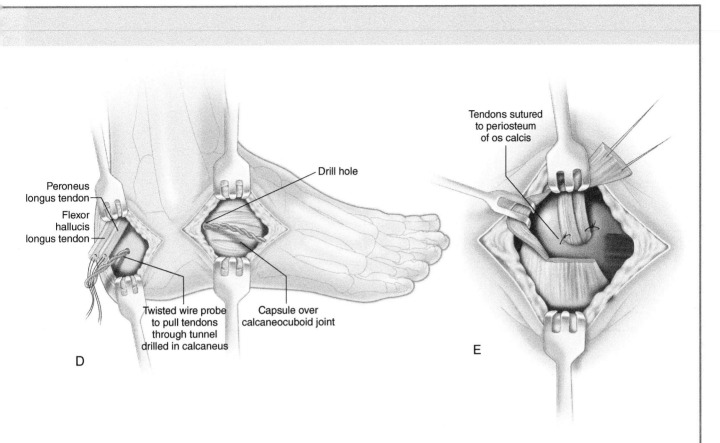

D, Through a lateral incision, the intermuscular septum is widely divided between the lateral and posterior compartments. An Ober tendon passer is inserted through the wound and directed anterior to the Achilles tendon into the transverse incision over the os calcis. The threads of the whip sutures at the ends of the peroneal tendons are passed through the hole in the tendon passer and the tendons are delivered at the heel. The posterior tibial tendon is delivered at the heel by a similar route, through an incision in the intermuscular septum between the medial and posterior compartments and anterior to the Achilles tendon. Next,

with a twisted wire probe, the tendons are inserted into the hole and pulled through the tunnel in the calcaneus.

E, At their point of exit on the lateral aspect of the calcaneus the tendons are sutured to the periosteum and ligamentous tissues. The tendons are sutured under enough tension to hold the foot in 15 degrees of equinus when the remaining ankle dorsiflexors are fair in motor strength and in 30 degrees of equinus if they are good or normal. The tendons are sutured to each other and to the periosteum of the apophysis of the calcaneus at the posterior end of the tunnel.

Continued on following page

Procedure 32 Posterior Tendon Transfer to the Os Calcis for Correction of Calcaneus Deformity (Green and Grice Procedure), cont'd

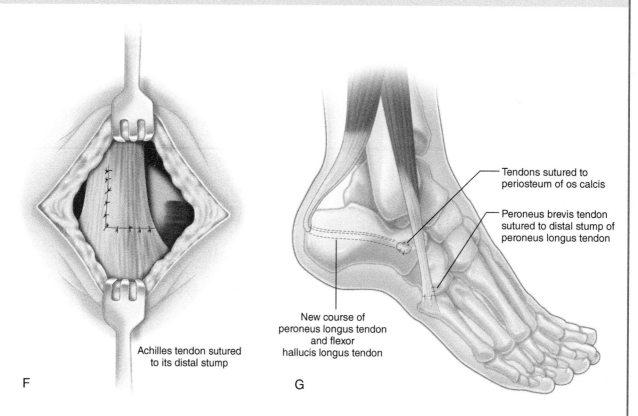

Achilles tendon sutured
to its distal stump

F

Tendons sutured to
periosteum of os calcis

Peroneus brevis tendon
sutured to distal stump of
peroneus longus tendon

New course of
peroneus longus tendon
and flexor
hallucis longus tendon

G

F and **G,** The divided portion of the Achilles tendon is resutured in its original position posterior to the transferred tendons.

The wounds are closed and a long-leg cast is applied to hold the knee in 45 to 60 degrees of flexion and the hindfoot in 15 to 30 degrees equinus, but the forefoot in neutral position. Cavus deformity of the forefoot should be avoided.

Postoperative Care

Three to 4 weeks after surgery the solid cast is removed and a new above-knee bivalved cast is made to protect the limb at all times when exercises are not being performed. It is imperative to prevent forced dorsiflexion of the ankle and stretching of the transferred tendons.

Exercises are first performed in the side-lying position with gravity eliminated and then in the prone position against gravity. To teach the patient the new action of the transferred muscle, the patient is asked to move the foot in the direction of a component of the original action of the muscle and then to plantar flex the foot. For example, when the peroneals are transferred, the patient is asked to evert and plantar flex the foot or, when the anterior tibial is transferred, to invert and plantar flex the foot. Soon, under supervision, guided dorsiflexion of the foot is performed along with plantar flexion. It is important to develop reciprocal motion and motor strength of the agonistic and antagonistic muscles. Weight bearing is not allowed. Ambulation is permitted in an above-knee bivalved cast with crutches.

In about 4 to 6 weeks, when the transferred tendons are fair in motor strength, the patient is allowed to stand on both feet. The heel of the foot that was operated on rests on a 3-cm-thick block to prevent stretching of the transferred tendons. Bearing partial weight on the foot, the patient should rise up on tiptoes while holding onto a table with the hands or using two crutches.

When the transplant functions effectively during tiptoe standing, walking with crutches is begun with three-point gait and partial weight bearing on the affected limb. The heel of the shoe is elevated with a 1- to 1.5-cm lift that tapers in front (toward the toes). Walking periods are gradually increased. When the transplant works effectively in gait and take-off has been developed in walking, standing-tiptoe rising exercises are started without the support of crutches. The knee should not be flexed and the patient should not lean forward while rising up on the toes at least three times. This may take a long time (as much as a year or more), but it is an important phase of postoperative management.

A plantar flexion spring orthosis or an orthosis with posterior elastic is worn when the patient is uncooperative in the use of crutches or when muscular control of the knee and hip is poor because of extensive paralysis. A stop at the ankle prevents dorsiflexion of the ankle beyond neutral position.

Procedure 33   Triple Arthrodesis

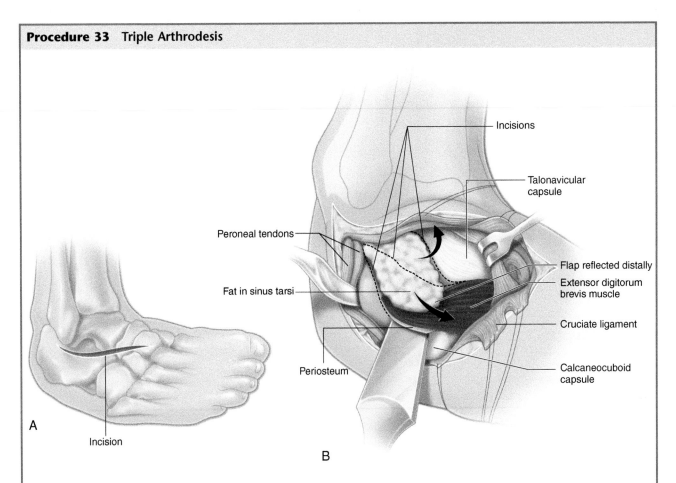

A, Incision

B,

- Incisions
- Talonavicular capsule
- Peroneal tendons
- Fat in sinus tarsi
- Flap reflected distally
- Extensor digitorum brevis muscle
- Cruciate ligament
- Periosteum
- Calcaneocuboid capsule

Operative Technique

A pneumatic tourniquet is placed on the proximal aspect of the thigh, and the patient is positioned semilaterally with a large sandbag under the hip on the affected side.
A, A curvilinear incision centered over the sinus tarsi is made. It starts one fingerbreadth distal and posterior to the tip of the lateral malleolus and extends anteriorly and distally to the base of the second metatarsal bone.
B, Skin flaps should not be developed. The incision is carried to the floor of the sinus tarsi. By sharp dissection with scalpel and periosteal elevator, the periosteum of the calcaneus, the adipose tissue contents of the sinus tarsi, and the tendinous origin of the extensor digitorum brevis

are elevated in one mass from the calcaneus and lateral aspect of the neck of the talus and retracted distally. It is essential to provide a viable soft tissue pedicle to obliterate the dead space remaining at the end of the operation.

Next an incision is made superiorly over the periosteum of the talus, and the head and neck of the talus are carefully exposed. The upper flap of the skin, subcutaneous tissue, and periosteum should be kept as thick as possible to avoid necrosis. Traction sutures are placed on the periosteum. At no time are the skin edges to be retracted. It is not necessary to divide the peroneal tendons or their sheaths. By subperiosteal dissection, the peroneal tendons are retracted posteriorly to expose the subtalar joint.

Continued on following page

Procedure 33   Triple Arthrodesis, cont'd

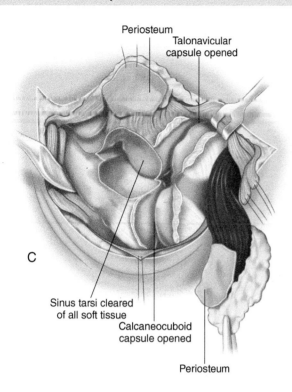

Periosteum

Talonavicular capsule opened

C

Sinus tarsi cleared of all soft tissue

Calcaneocuboid capsule opened

Periosteum

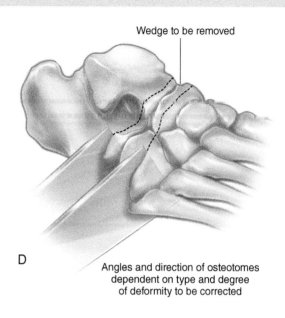

Wedge to be removed

D

Angles and direction of osteotomes dependent on type and degree of deformity to be corrected

C and **D,** The capsules of the calcaneocuboid, talonavicular, and subtalar joints are incised. These joints are opened and their cartilaginous surfaces clearly visualized by turning the foot into varus position. A lamina spreader placed in the sinus tarsi will aid in exposure of the posterior subtalar joint. Before excision of the articular cartilaginous surfaces, the surgeon should review the deformity of the foot and decide on the wedges of bone to be removed for correction of the deformity. Circulation of the talus and the complications of avascular necrosis of the talus and arthritis of the ankle after triple arthrodesis should always be kept in mind. The height of the foot is another consideration. A low lateral malleolus causes difficulty wearing shoes. At times, it is best to add a bone graft rather than resect wedges of bone. With a sharp osteotome, the cartilaginous surfaces of the calcaneocuboid joint are excised. Next the articular cartilage surface of the talonavicular joint is exposed, the plane of osteotomy being perpendicular to the long axis of the neck of the talus and parallel to the calcaneocuboid joint. When the beak of the navicular is unduly prominent medially or when, in a varus foot, one cannot obtain adequate exposure of the talonavicular joint without excessive retraction, a second dorsomedial incision may be used to expose the talonavicular joint.

E to H, With a lamina spreader in the sinus tarsi, the subtalar joint is widely exposed and the cartilage of the anterior and posterior joints is excised. The surgeon should keep in mind the neurovascular structures behind the medial malleolus. The wedges of bone that must be removed to correct the deformity are excised in one mass with the articular cartilage. It is of great help to leave the osteotome used on the opposing articular surface in place and held steady by the assistant as a second osteotome or gouge is used to take contiguous cartilage and bone. The divided articular surfaces of the joints to undergo arthrodesis are fish-scaled for maximum raw cancellous bony contact.

The skin is closed with interrupted sutures. A well-molded long-leg cast is applied with the foot held in the desired position. We have not found fixation of the joints by staples necessary and do not recommend it. In foot stabilization in children with cerebral palsy, especially in the severely athetoid or spastic child, secure crisscross Kirschner wires are used to maintain position. These wires are removed in 6 to 8 weeks.

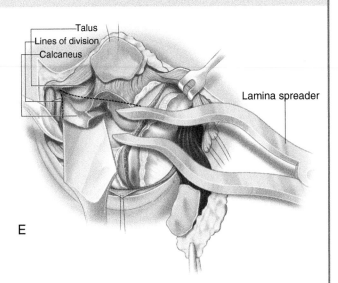

E

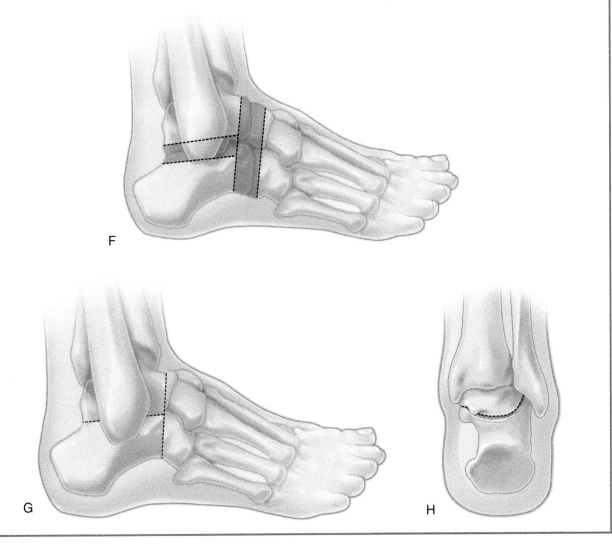

F

G

H

Procedure 34   Extraarticular Arthrodesis of the Subtalar Joint (Grice Procedure)

Operative Technique

A, A 2-in-long, slightly curved incision is made over the subtalar joint, centered over the sinus tarsi.

B, The incision is carried down to the sinus tarsi. The capsules of the posterior and anterior subtalar articulations are identified and left intact. The operation is extraarticular. If the capsule is opened inadvertently, it should be closed with interrupted sutures.

The periosteum on the talus corresponding to the lateral margin of the roof of the sinus tarsi is divided and reflected proximally. The fibrofatty tissue in the sinus tarsi along with the periosteum of the calcaneus corresponding to the floor of the sinus tarsi and the tendinous origin of the short toe extensors from the calcaneus are elevated and reflected distally in one mass.

C, The remaining fatty and ligamentous tissue from the sinus tarsi is thoroughly removed with a sharp scalpel and curet.

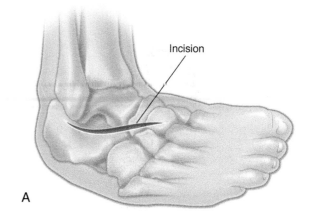

Incision

A

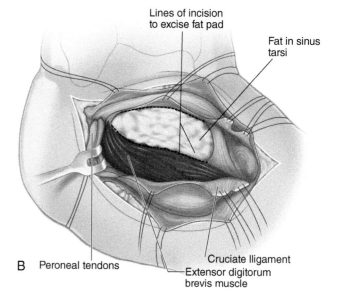

Lines of incision to excise fat pad

Fat in sinus tarsi

B   Peroneal tendons

Cruciate lligament
Extensor digitorum brevis muscle

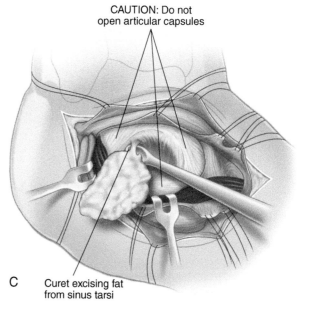

CAUTION: Do not open articular capsules

C   Curet excising fat from sinus tarsi

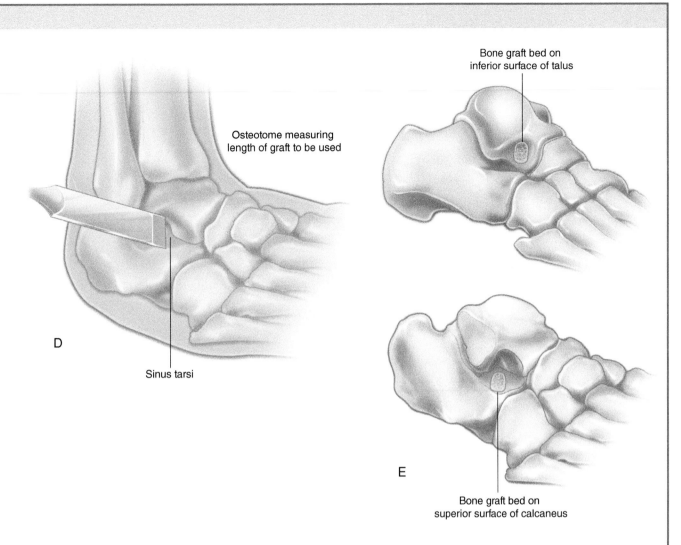

Osteotome measuring
length of graft to be used

D

Sinus tarsi

Bone graft bed on
inferior surface of talus

E

Bone graft bed on
superior surface of calcaneus

D, Next the foot is manipulated into equinus position and inversion and the calcaneus rotated into its normal position beneath the talus to correct the valgus deformity. Broad straight osteotomes of various size (¾ to 1¼ in or more) are inserted into the sinus tarsi to block the subtalar joint and determine the length and optimum position of the bone graft and the stability that it will provide. The long axis of the graft should be parallel to that of the leg when the ankle is dorsiflexed into neutral position, and the hindfoot should be in 5 degrees valgus or neutral, but never varus. Even a slight degree of varus deformity of the heel seems to increase with growth.

E, The optimal site of the bone graft bed is marked with the broad osteotome. A thin layer of cortical bone (⅛ to ⅟₁₆ in) is removed with a dental osteotome from the inferior surface of the talus (the roof of the sinus tarsi) and the superior surface of the calcaneus (the floor of the sinus tarsi) at the site marked for the bone graft. It is best to preserve the most lateral cortical margin of the graft bed to support the bone block and prevent it from sinking into soft cancellous bone.

Continued on following page

Procedure 34   Extraarticular Arthrodesis of the Subtalar Joint (Grice Procedure), cont'd

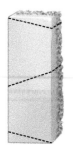
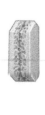

Shaping of bone graft
from tibia

Shaped fibular graft
(our preferred method)

F

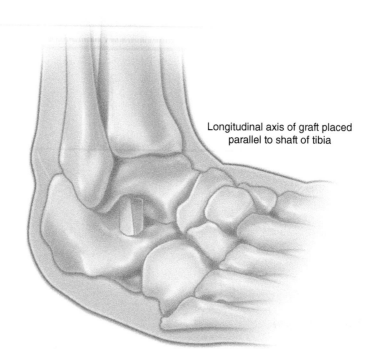

Longitudinal axis of graft placed
parallel to shaft of tibia

F, A bone graft of appropriate size can be taken from the anteromedial surface of the proximal tibial metaphysis as a single cortical graft, which is then cut into two trapezoidal bone grafts with their cancellous surfaces facing each other. We prefer to use fibular bone grafts with the cortices intact. The corners of the base of the graft are removed with a rongeur so that it is trapezoidal and can be countersunk into cancellous bone and thereby prevent lateral displacement after surgery.

The bone graft is placed in the prepared graft bed in the sinus tarsi by holding the foot in varus position. An impactor may be used to fix the cortices of the graft in place. The longitudinal axis of the graft should be parallel to the shaft of the tibia with the ankle in neutral position.

With the foot held in the desired position, the distal soft tissue pedicle of fibrofatty tissue of the sinus tarsi, the calcaneal periosteum, and the tendinous origin of the short toe extensors are sutured to the reflected periosteum from the talus. The subcutaneous tissue and skin are closed with interrupted sutures, and an above-knee cast is applied.

Postoperative Care

The cast is removed 6 to 10 weeks after surgery and radiographs are taken. If there is solid healing of the graft, gradual weight bearing is allowed with the protection of crutches. Active and passive exercises are performed to strengthen the muscles and increase range of motion of the ankle and knee.

Procedure 35 Extensor Carpi Ulnaris—Extensor Carpi Radialis Brevis Transfer

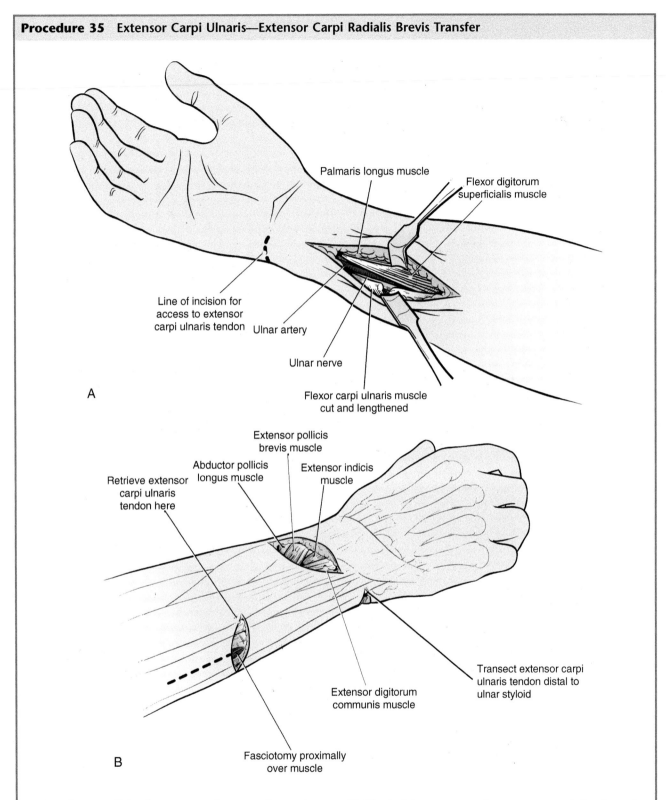

Palmaris longus muscle

Flexor digitorum superficialis muscle

Line of incision for access to extensor carpi ulnaris tendon

Ulnar artery

Ulnar nerve

Flexor carpi ulnaris muscle cut and lengthened

A

Extensor pollicis brevis muscle

Abductor pollicis longus muscle

Extensor indicis muscle

Retrieve extensor carpi ulnaris tendon here

Transect extensor carpi ulnaris tendon distal to ulnar styloid

Extensor digitorum communis muscle

Fasciotomy proximally over muscle

B

A, Lengthening of the flexor carpi ulnaris tendon is done at the musculotendinous level in the distal part of the forearm. Lengthening of the other wrist flexors can be accomplished through the same incision if needed.

B, The incision to expose the extensor carpi ulnaris tendon is made just distal to the ulnar styloid. The extensor carpi ulnaris tendon is then retrieved into the proximal incision and transferred subcutaneously to the dorsoradial wrist incision.

Continued on following page

Procedure 35   Extensor Carpi Ulnaris—Extensor Carpi Radialis Brevis Transfer, cont'd

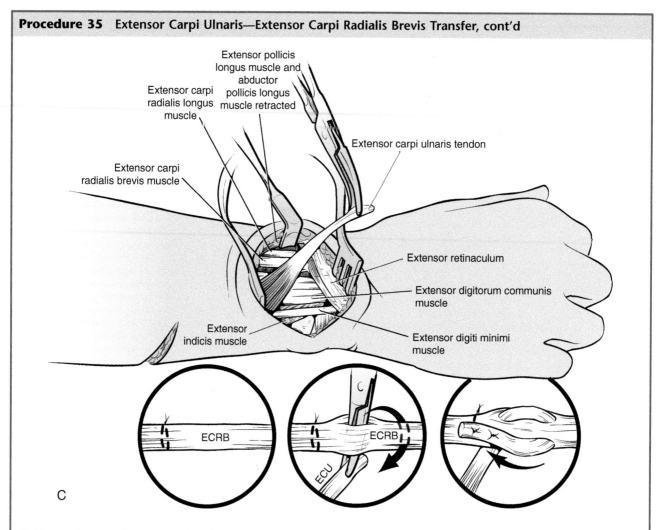

Extensor pollicis longus muscle and abductor pollicis longus muscle retracted

Extensor carpi radialis longus muscle

Extensor carpi radialis brevis muscle

Extensor carpi ulnaris tendon

Extensor retinaculum

Extensor digitorum communis muscle

Extensor indicis muscle

Extensor digiti minimi muscle

ECRB

ECRB

ECU

C

C, The tendon transfer is secured with a weave technique. The first suture is placed proximal to the site of the first pass of the donor tendon through the recipient tendon to prevent proximal migration of the tendon placement.

Procedure 36   Fractional Lengthening of the Finger and Wrist Flexors in the Forearm Operative Technique

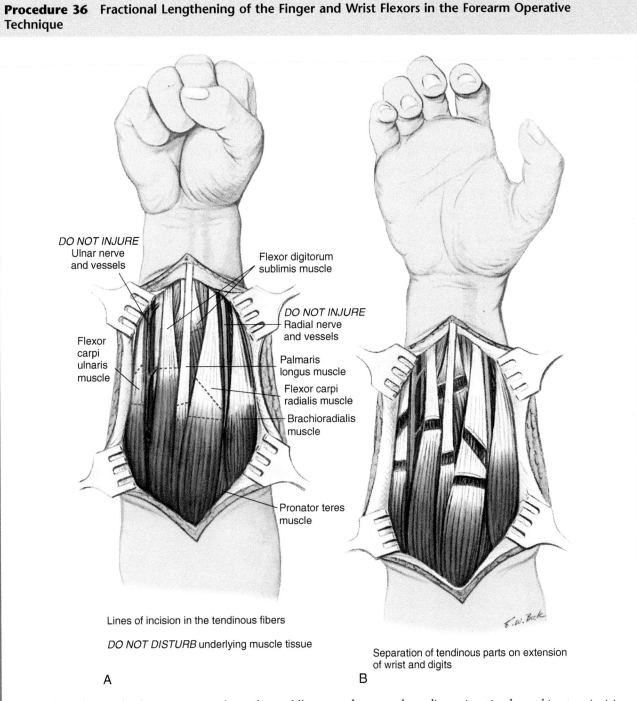

DO NOT INJURE
Ulnar nerve
and vessels

Flexor digitorum
sublimis muscle

DO NOT INJURE
Radial nerve
and vessels

Flexor
carpi
ulnaris
muscle

Palmaris
longus muscle

Flexor carpi
radialis muscle

Brachioradialis
muscle

Pronator teres
muscle

Lines of incision in the tendinous fibers

DO NOT DISTURB underlying muscle tissue

Separation of tendinous parts on extension
of wrist and digits

A

B

A, A midline longitudinal incision is made in the middle three fourths of the volar surface of the forearm. The subcutaneous tissue and deep fascia are divided in line with the skin incision. The wound flaps are undermined, elevated, and retracted with four-prong rake retractors to expose the superficial groups of muscles. On the radial side of the flexor carpi ulnaris tendon, the ulnar vessels and nerves are identified and protected from injury; similarly, on the radial side of the flexor carpi radialis tendon, the radial vessels and nerve are isolated to protect them from inadvertent damage. Sliding lengthening of the flexor carpi radialis and flexor carpi ulnaris muscles is performed at the musculotendinous junction by making two incisions in their tendinous fibers, about 1.5 cm apart, without disturbing the underlying muscle tissue. The proximal incision is transverse and the distal one is oblique. The palmaris longus and flexor digitorum muscles are lengthened by only one transverse incision in each.

B, The wrist and the fingers are passively hyperextended. The tendinous parts will separate, whereas the intact underlying muscle fibers will maintain continuity of the muscles.

Continued on following page

Procedure 36 Fractional Lengthening of the Finger and Wrist Flexors in the Forearm Operative Technique, cont'd

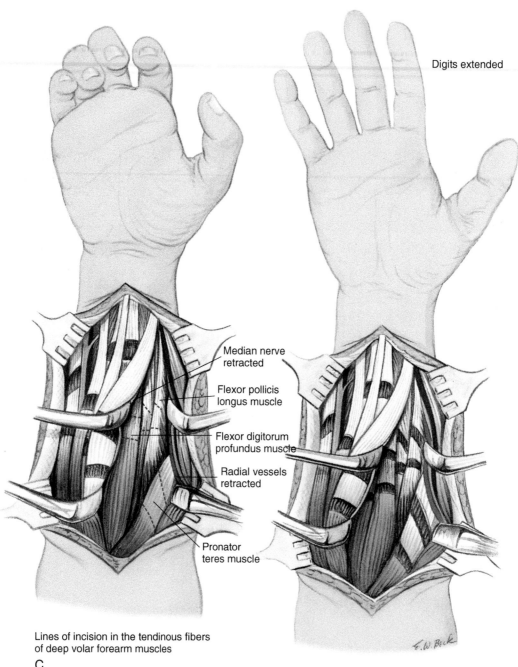

Digits extended

Median nerve retracted

Flexor pollicis longus muscle

Flexor digitorum profundus muscle

Radial vessels retracted

Pronator teres muscle

Lines of incision in the tendinous fibers of deep volar forearm muscles

C

Note the sliding lengthening by separation of tendinous fibers

D

C and D, The deep volar muscles are exposed by retracting the brachioradialis muscle and radial vessels radially and the flexor carpi radialis and flexor digitorum sublimis muscles ulnarward. The median nerve is identified and protected from injury by retracting it medially with the flexor carpi radialis muscle. The flexor pollicis longus and flexor digitorum profundus muscles are lengthened by making two incisions in their tendinous parts and sliding them in the same manner as described for the superficial volar forearm muscles. Continuity of muscles is maintained by gentle handling of tissues and by taking care that adequate muscle substance underlies the divided tendinous parts. Sliding lengthening is achieved by separating the tendinous fibers by slow, but firm extension of the thumb and four ulnar digits.

Next, the range of passive supination of the forearm is tested. If a pronation contracture is present, the pronator teres muscle is lengthened by two oblique incisions, 1.5 cm apart, in its tendinous fibers. Again, the underlying muscle tissue should not be disturbed. The forearm is forcibly supinated; the tendinous segments will slide and separate, thereby elongating the muscle.

The tourniquet is released and complete hemostasis is obtained. The deep fascia is not closed. The subcutaneous tissue and skin are approximated by interrupted sutures. An above-elbow cast that includes all the fingers and the thumb is applied to immobilize the forearm in full supination, the elbow in 90 degrees of flexion, the wrist in 50 degrees of extension, and the fingers and thumb in neutral extension.

Postoperative Care

Four weeks after surgery, the cast is removed and active exercises are started to develop motor power in the elongated muscle. Squeezing soft balls of various size and other functional exercises are carried out several times a day. An aggressive occupational therapy program is essential. The corrected position is maintained in a bivalved cast. As motor function develops in the elongated muscle and its antagonists, periods out of the cast are gradually increased.

Procedure 37   **Scapulocostal Stabilization for Scapular Winging (Ketenjian Technique)**

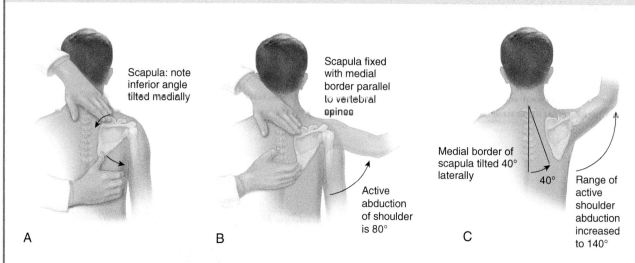

In winging of the scapula in patients with facioscapulo-humeral muscular dystrophy, the scapula is malrotated, with its longitudinal axis deviated medially and its inferomedial angle displaced toward the spinous process of the vertebrae.

Preoperative Assessment

Before surgery, the surgeon must determine the position in which the scapula will be fixed to the thoracic wall. This is done with the patient standing and the surgeon behind the patient.
A, The surgeon steadies the scapula with one hand by holding its superomedial border with the thumb and fingers. With the thumb of the opposite hand, the surgeon hooks the inferior angle of the scapula while the palm and fingers grasp the thoracic cage laterally. The patient's arm hangs loosely at the side.

B, The inferior angle of the scapula is displaced laterally until the medial border of the scapula is parallel to the longitudinal axis of the spinous processes of the vertebrae. With the scapula fixed on the thoracic cage, the patient actively abducts the shoulder, and the degree of glenohumeral active abduction is measured. In this illustration, active shoulder abduction is 80 degrees.
C, The inferior angle of the scapula is displaced laterally, thus rotating the scapula laterally in the coronal (scapular) plane. In this illustration the medial border of the scapula is tilted laterally 40 degrees in relation to the vertebral spines. The patient is asked to actively abduct the shoulder, and the total range of thoracoglenohumeral abduction is measured and correlated with the scapuloaxial angle (the angle formed by the medial border of the scapula and a longitudinal line connecting the spinous processes of the vertebrae).

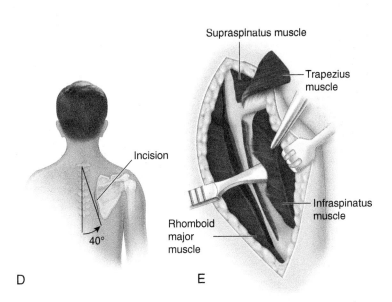

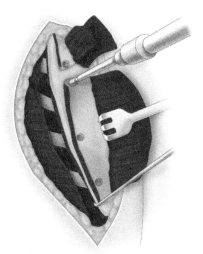

Drill holes made 1.3 cm
from medial border of scapula

F

Operative Technique

At surgery the scapula is fixed to the thoracic cage at the scapuloaxial angle measured during the maximum desired position of shoulder abduction. The operation is performed with the patient prone. The neck, entire thorax, and involved upper limb are prepared and carefully draped to allow free manipulation of the shoulder.

D, With the scapula in position to be fixed to the thoracic cage, a longitudinal incision is made at its medial border. The subcutaneous tissue and superficial fascia are divided in line with the skin incision.

E, The trapezius, levator scapulae, and rhomboids are sectioned from the medial border of the scapula; these muscles are atrophic and have been replaced by fibrous or fibrofatty tissue. The supraspinatus, infraspinatus, and subscapularis are elevated with a periosteal elevator for a distance of 2.5 cm from the medial border of the scapula.

F, Four drill holes are made 1.3 cm from the medial border of the scapula at the level of the adjacent ribs when the scapula is placed in the desired position for stabilization. The scapula is tilted to approximately 20 degrees of lateral rotation.

G, The ribs underlying the drill holes in the scapula are exposed subperiosteally. The surgeon must be extremely careful to not injure the intercostal vessels and

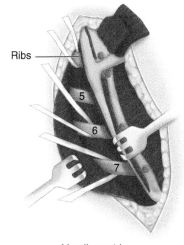

Mersilene strips
passed around ribs

G

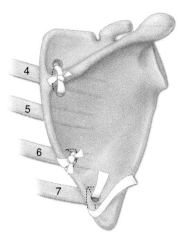

Strips pulled through drill holes
and tied down snugly with scapula
positioned in 40° external rotation

H

nerves at the inferior margin of the ribs. Mersilene or fasciae latae strips are then passed around the ribs.

H, The strips are passed through drill holes and tied snugly with the scapula maintained in 20 degrees of lateral rotation. The stability of the scapula's fixation to the rib cage is tested, and the wound is closed in the usual fashion.

Postoperative Care

The upper limb is supported in a sling. Several days postoperatively, active assisted and gentle passive range-of-motion exercises are performed several times a day. Codman pendulum exercises are begun 7 days after surgery. The sling support is discontinued 4 to 5 weeks after the operation.

SECTION III

SPINE DISORDERS

The technique of rigid segmental fixation of the spine using pedicle screws as anchors has given the surgeon the ability to gain often dramatic deformity correction of spinal deformities. Great care is required, including neurophysiologic spinal cord monitoring, to avoid injury to the spinal cord itself or to its blood supply. Failures of fusion are rare, and patients return to activity quite quickly. Anterior techniques are used infrequently today but are occasionally needed. Lumbar or thoracolumbar kyphectomy is a demanding procedure and is usually done in centers specializing in neuromuscular conditions. Pelvic fixation is often necessary for neurogenic scoliosis to maintain overall pelvic balance.

Procedure 38   Exposure of the Spine for Posterior Instrumentation and Fusion

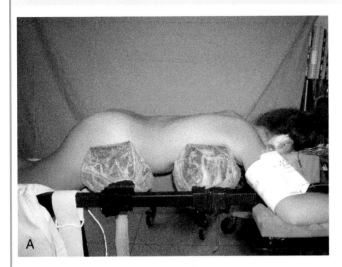

A

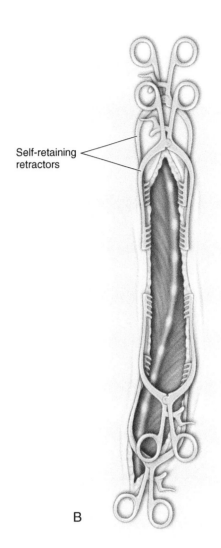

Self-retaining retractors

B

Operative Technique

General anesthesia is administered via endotracheal intubation. Intravenous access is obtained, followed by placement of a radial arterial line. Perioperative antibiotics, usually first-generation cephalosporins, are administered. **A,** *Positioning the patient.* Under the supervision of the surgeon, the patient is placed prone on an OSI frame. Gel pads may be placed over the four support pads to further cushion the chest and inguinal region. The abdomen is free of any contact to minimize blood loss. The upper pads rest on the upper part of the chest just lateral to the nipple region. The shoulders are abducted and the elbows are flexed. The axillae should be free of pressure, without stretching across the brachial plexus or pressure over the ulnar nerve (at the elbow). The lower pads make contact at the ilioinguinal region. Unless the lateral femoral cutaneous nerve is padded satisfactorily, pressure can lead to temporary postoperative dysesthesia in the anterior aspect of the thigh. When instrumented into the lumbar spine, the hips should be extended by elevating the legs with pillows placed under the anterior part of the thigh to ensure that lumbar lordosis is maintained.

The entire back is prepared with povidone-iodine (Betadine) or chlorhexidine, beginning at the base of the hairline and continuing to the gluteal cleft. Both iliac crests are included in the surgical field. After preparation and draping, a Betadine-impregnated, sticky drape is applied. An adequate area must be exposed so that the incision never extends to the edge of the drapes.

B, *Incision.* The length of the skin incision is determined by the number of levels requiring fusion. The incision is taken down to the dermis with a scalpel. To minimize bleeding, electrocautery is used to continue the incision down through the dermis into subcutaneous tissue. An alternative to this technique is to infiltrate the intradermal tissue with epinephrine and then sharply incise down to the subcutaneous tissue. Self-retaining retractors are next placed into the wound to keep the skin edges under tension and provide exposure of the spinous processes. (Although minimally invasive surgery has been attempted for adolescent idiopathic scoliosis, the results have not been widely reported and it probably does not have any significant advantages. Early reports suggest longer surgery and little benefit with respect to shorter hospital stays, and it is far too early to determine the incidence of pseudarthrosis, a significant risk given the limited exposure.)

Continued on following page

Procedure 38   Exposure of the Spine for Posterior Instrumentation and Fusion, cont'd

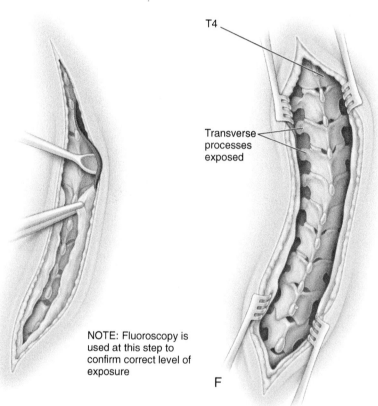

Cobb periosteal elevator reflecting cartilaginous caps to expose spinous processes on both sides

Incision of periosteum over spinous processes to bony tip

C

Interspinous ligament

D

NOTE: Subperiosteal stripping to facet joints begins distally and proceeds proximally in the thoracic spine

T4

Transverse processes exposed

NOTE: Fluoroscopy is used at this step to confirm correct level of exposure

E

F

C, Once the spinous processes have been exposed, the median raphe is incised sharply down to bone. A Kelly clamp may provide proper orientation for the incision. Dissection in this avascular plane minimizes blood loss.

D, Cobb elevators are used to subperiosteally expose the posterior elements. The exposure extends laterally to the tips of the transverse processes of all the levels included in the fusion. Meticulous dissection should be performed to prepare the posterior elements for fusion.

E, As the subperiosteal dissection continues, each level is packed firmly with gauze to minimize bleeding.

F, Once the dissection is completed, the packing is removed and self-retaining retractors are placed at the proximal, distal, and intermediate areas. Further cleaning of the surgical field is then performed with rongeurs, curets, and electrocautery.

Intraoperative fluoroscopy is used to confirm the proper levels for fusion. Regardless of the surgeon's expertise, fluoroscopy should always be performed to avoid inadvertent selection of the wrong vertebral level.

After exposure of the surgical field, anchor sites (hooks, wires, or screws) are prepared. Preoperative planning for proper hook and screw placement should be noted on the radiograph and should be familiar to all those assisting in the operation.

Procedure 39 Ponte Osteotomy

Operative Technique

A, After the posterior spine has been stripped of its para-spinal muscles, Ponte osteotomies can be completed either before or after pedicle screws are placed. The author prefers to perform the osteotomies after the screw tracts have been prepared for placement of screws to limit exposure to the spinal canal during the preparation of screws. The spinous processes are first partially excised with a Leksell rongeur. The ligamentum flavum is excised in the central most aspect until epidural fat is seen. A Kerrison rongeur is then used to remove the remaining ligamentum flavum as well as the superior and inferior articular facets. An alternative step is to perform inferior facetectomies in the normal method using a Capener gouge or straight osteotomies.

B, A side view of the spine demonstrating an intact spine *(left)* and following Ponte osteotomies at all levels *(right)*. Note the ability for these osteotomies to allow the spine to close posteriorly by hinging on the anterior and middle columns of the spine.

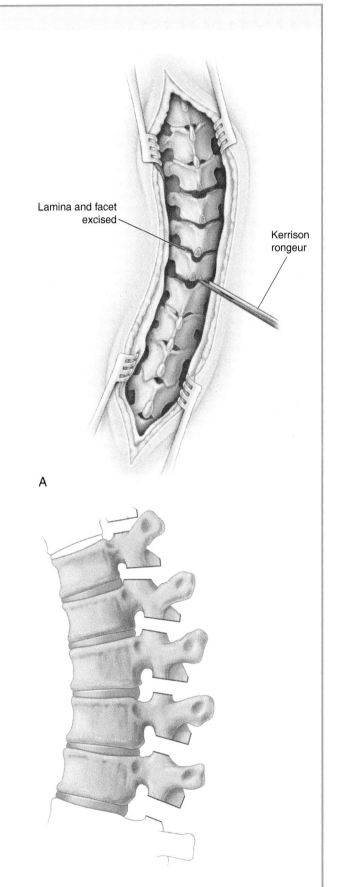

Lamina and facet excised

Kerrison rongeur

A

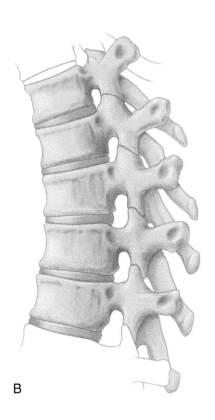

B

Procedure 40   Posterior Spinal Instrumentation and Fusion Using Pedicle Screws

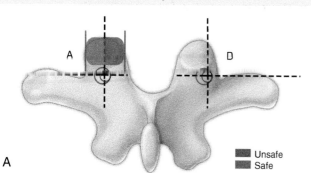

A

A, Safe placement of segmental pedicle screws is essential. The starting point must never be medial to the midpoint of the superior facet. (Redrawn from Medtronic Sofamor Danek USA, Inc., Memphis, Tenn, with permission.)
B, Using the straightforward approach, the thoracic vertebral cephalad–caudad starting points vary slightly depending on the levels being instrumented. *TP,* Transverse process. (Redrawn from Medtronic Sofamor Danek USA, Inc. Memphis, Tenn, with permission.)

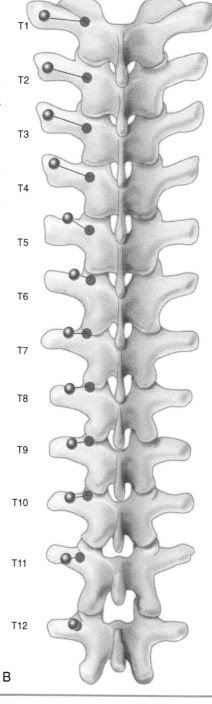

■ Unsafe
■ Safe

Level	Cephalad-Caudad Starting Point
T1	Midpoint TP
T2	Midpoint TP
T3	Midpoint TP
T4	Proximal third TP
T5	Proximal third TP
T6	Proximal third TP
T7	Proximal TP
T8	Proximal TP
T9	Proximal TP
T10	Junction: Proximal edge–proximal third TP
T11	Proximal third TP
T12	Midpoint TP

B

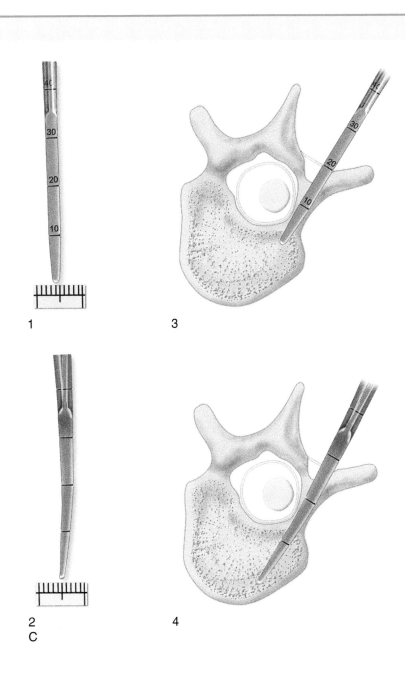

1

3

2
C

4

C, *1* and *2*: Preparation for the pedicle screw sites should begin at the most distal vertebra to be instrumented and proceed cephalad. Either the freehand technique or the fluoroscopy-guided technique can be used. A thoracic gearshift (2-mm blunt-tipped curved pedicle finder) is used to enter the pedicle.

3: To avoid medial wall penetration, the gearshift is initially pointed laterally when the pedicle is entered.

4: After insertion to 15 to 20 mm, the pedicle finder is reversed (medial orientation) to continue penetration into the vertebral body to a depth approximating 30 to 40 mm, depending on the vertebra level. Once this is accomplished, a ball-tipped probe is used to palpate all four walls of the pedicle and the floor (anterior vertebral body). The depth that is measured will approximate the screw length that will be needed. (From Kim YJ, Lenke LG, Bridwell KH, et al: Free hand pedicle screw placement in the thoracic spine: is it safe? *Spine* 29:333, 2004.)

Continued on following page

Procedure 40   Posterior Spinal Instrumentation and Fusion Using Pedicle Screws, cont'd

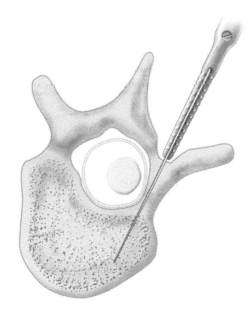

1

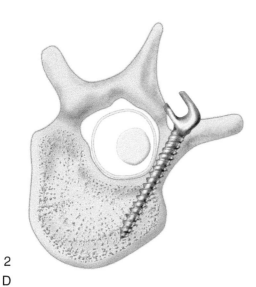

2

D

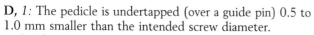

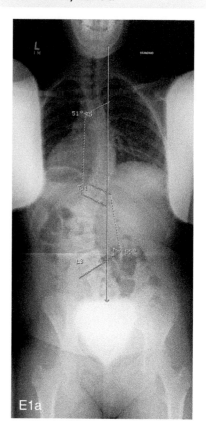

E1a

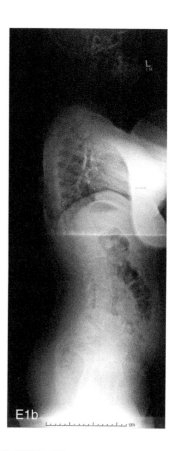

E1b

D, 1: The pedicle is undertapped (over a guide pin) 0.5 to 1.0 mm smaller than the intended screw diameter.

   2: The screw is then slowly inserted freehand.
E, All screws are placed.

   1a and *1b:* Preoperative anteroposterior (AP) and lateral radiographs of a Lenke 6C curve.

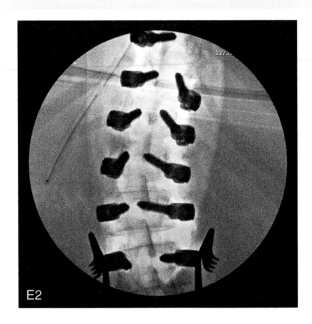

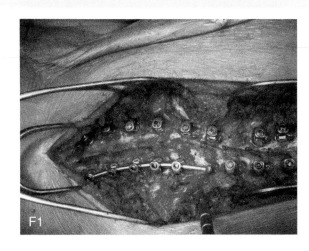

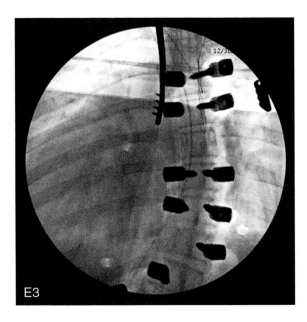

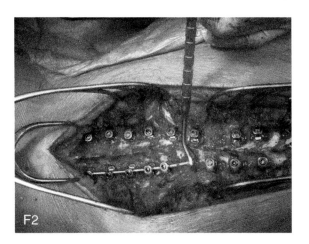

F, 1: A precontoured provisional convex right lumbar rod is placed.

   2: Following rod rotation of the lumbar provisional right rod.

   2: Fluoroscopic images demonstrating accurate placement of the lumbar screws.

   3: Lumbar screws.

Continued on following page

Procedure 40   Posterior Spinal Instrumentation and Fusion Using Pedicle Screws, cont'd

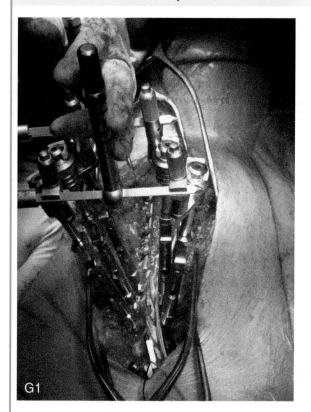

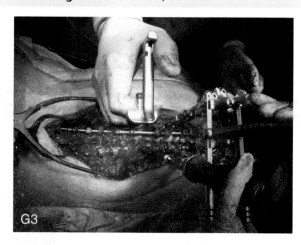

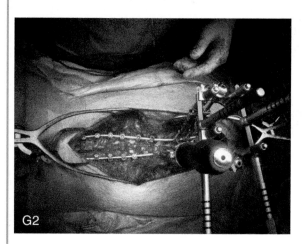

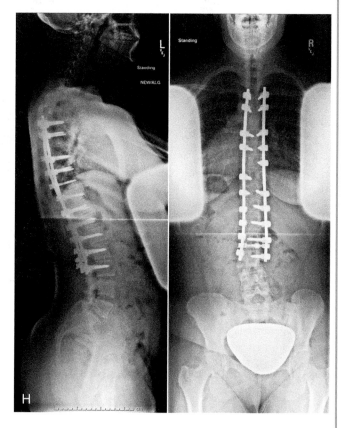

G, *1:* The left final rod with a precontour is placed with the right thoracic kyphosis and left lumbar lordosis while the provisional right lumbar rod is in place.

2: An apical derotation maneuver is performed via the en bloc rotation technique with the left rod in place.

3: The left rod is in place.

H, Final AP and lateral radiographs at 2 years after surgery demonstrating good correction in the AP and lateral planes.

Procedure 41   Sacro-Iliac Screws

Fixation of the spinal instrumentation construct to the pelvis is often necessary in neuromuscular scoliosis as well as other conditions which involve pelvic obliquity. The technique described is currently preferred for its low profile and stable fixation.

Operative Technique

After stripping the muscle off the posterior sacrum, the first and second sacral dorsal foramen are identified. **A,** The starting point is made half way between these two foramen along an imaginary line on the lateral aspect of

the foramen. The awl is then directed inferiorly 40 to 50 degrees relative to a horizontal line connecting the posterior superior iliac spine and 20 to 30 degrees caudal from a straight lateral projection. **B,** The awl is advanced under fluoroscopic guidance in the AP projection to ensure a true orthogonal view is being obtained. **C,** The awl should be directed so it is just lateral and anterior to the sciatic notch for optimum fixation. The AP view demonstrating a well-placed screw. **D,** A fluoroscopic view shooting straight down the screw demonstrates the screw between the inner and outer cortices of the ilium, and the teardrop is seen with the screw in the center.

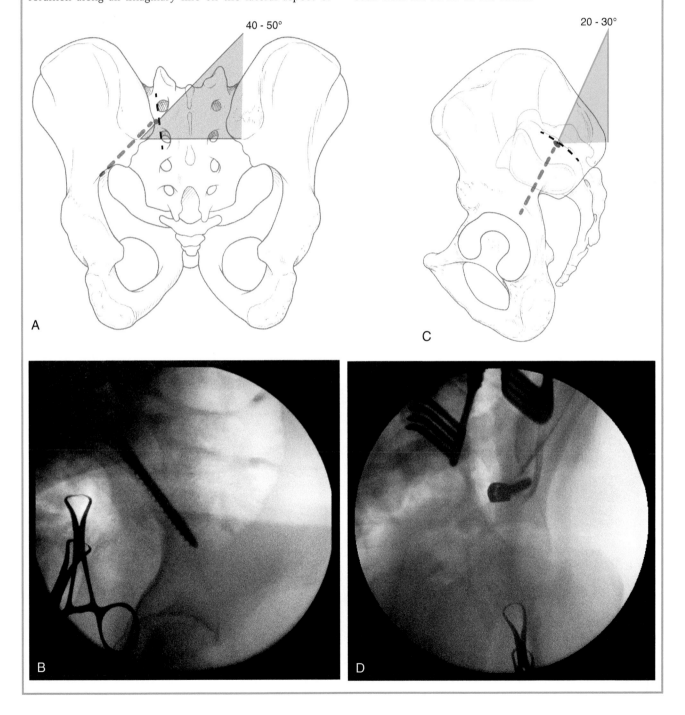

Procedure 42   Anterior Instrumentation of the Spine for Thoracolumbar or Lumbar Scoliosis

Incision

Cut line at
costocartilage angle

Incision
(along path of 10th rib)

Spinous process of T10

B

Periosteal bed of
resected 10th rib

Sutures are
placed prior
to splitting
of cartilage

C

10th rib cartilage
is split with scalpel

A

Operative Technique

In this plate the thoracoabdominal approach for exposure of the lower thoracic and lumbar spine is described.

A, *Positioning.* Under the direction of the surgeon, the patient is placed in the lateral decubitus position (the convexity of the curve is upward). A roll is placed under the axilla of the dependent arm. The body is supported with a deflatable beanbag. The upper part of the arm is flexed forward and slightly abducted. The operating table may be temporarily flexed (at the apex of the scoliosis) to facilitate excision of the intervertebral disks.

Approach. It will be necessary to remove a rib for exposure of the spine. Ideally, the rib that is removed is the one immediately cephalad to the uppermost vertebral body requiring instrumentation. For instrumentation between T11 and L3, removal of the tenth rib allows adequate exposure.

Skin incision. The incision begins lateral to the spinous process of T10 (or T9) and extends along the course of the tenth rib to the costocartilaginous junction and then across the upper part of the abdomen to the lateral edge of the rectus abdominis. Here, it turns distally toward the symphysis pubis and stops at the level of the umbilicus.

B, The tenth rib is freed subperiosteally, divided at its costocartilaginous junction, and removed. This creates a larger working aperture and provides a source of autogenous bone graft.

C, Once the costal cartilage of the tenth rib is split, the retroperitoneal space is identified and entered.

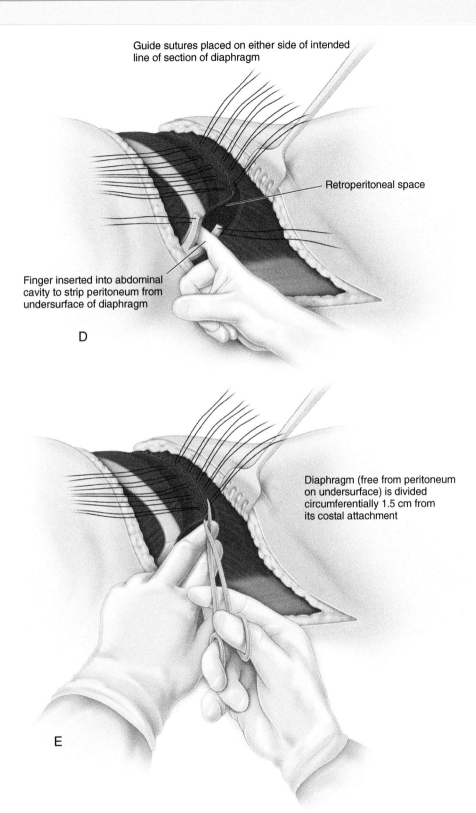

Guide sutures placed on either side of intended line of section of diaphragm

Retroperitoneal space

Finger inserted into abdominal cavity to strip peritoneum from undersurface of diaphragm

D

Diaphragm (free from peritoneum on undersurface) is divided circumferentially 1.5 cm from its costal attachment

E

D, Using blunt finger dissection, the operator separates the peritoneum from the inferior aspect of the diaphragm. Once freed, the viscera lie safely away from the vertebral bodies. Identification sutures are placed on either side of the intended line of division of the diaphragm, which is ½ to ¾ inch from its periphery. Placement of several of these sutures facilitates proper closure of the diaphragm later.
E, The diaphragm is sectioned from its costal attachments.

Continued on following page

Procedure 42 Anterior Instrumentation of the Spine for Thoracolumbar or Lumbar Scoliosis, cont'd

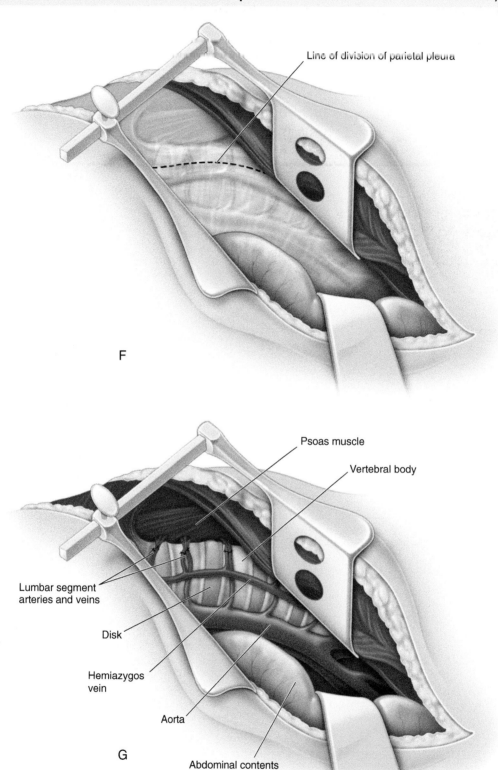

Line of division of parietal pleura

F

Psoas muscle

Vertebral body

Lumbar segment
arteries and veins

Disk

Hemiazygos
vein

Aorta

G

Abdominal contents
retracted

F, Next, the parietal pleura is incised along the thoracic vertebral bodies that are to be included in the fusion.
G, In the lumbar region, the psoas muscle is gently elevated off the vertebral bodies and intervertebral disks and retracted posteriorly. The segmental vessels are ligated in the middle of each vertebral body included in the fusion. The aorta and vena cava are protected with retractors, and the anterior longitudinal ligament is partially excised with a sharp scalpel. Each disk within the levels selected for fusion is removed with various rongeurs and curets.

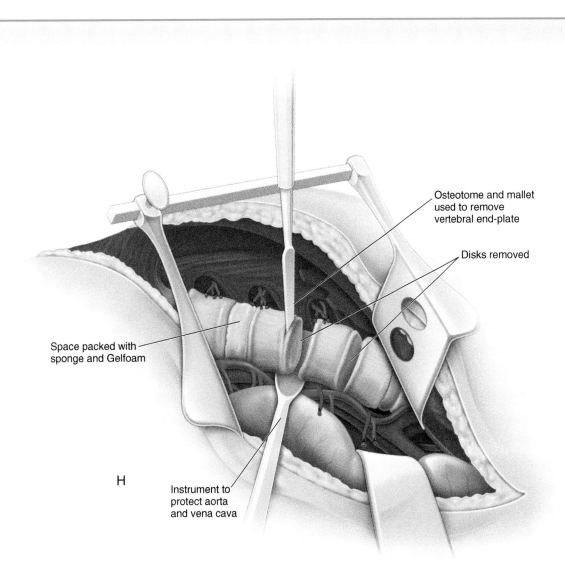

Osteotome and mallet
used to remove
vertebral end-plate

Disks removed

Space packed with
sponge and Gelfoam

H

Instrument to
protect aorta
and vena cava

H, With a curet or sharp osteotome and mallet, the operator removes the vertebral cartilaginous end-plates and retained pieces of disk. For correction of kyphosis, most of the annular ligamentous tissue down to the posterior longitudinal ligament is removed. For scoliosis, however, the outer annular fibers need not be fully removed. The disk spaces are then temporarily packed with Gelfoam to minimize bleeding. If the operating table was flexed to facilitate excision of intervertebral disks, it should be flattened at this time.

Continued on following page

Procedure 42   Anterior Instrumentation of the Spine for Thoracolumbar or Lumbar Scoliosis, cont'd

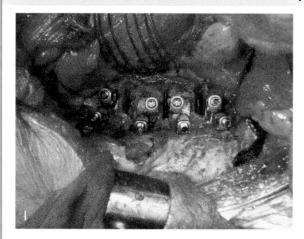

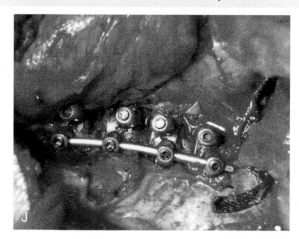

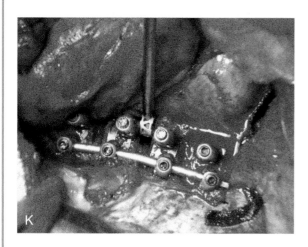

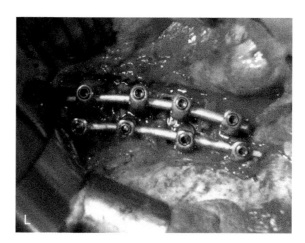

I, Following complete disk excision, the dual screws are placed via some guidance with a dual-headed staple. Retraction of the abdominal contents is seen at the top of the photo.

J, The precontoured posterior rod has been placed and a rod rotation maneuver was performed to correct the scoliosis and improve the lumbar lordosis.

K, Following rod rotation, anterior structural support is placed to maintain the lumbar lordosis, to assist in correction of the coronal plane deformity, and to increase the stiffness of the construct.

L, Final construct after the anterior rod has been placed.

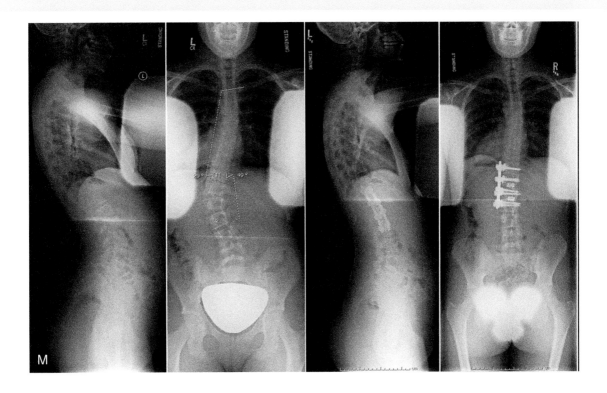

M, Preoperative and 2-year radiographs following anterior spinal fusion and instrumentation with a dual-rod system and anterior autologous rib bone graft.

SECTION IV

LOWER EXTREMITY DISORDERS

The Green modification of the Phemister technique for epiphseodesis is a time-honored, thorough method. Currently most surgeons use either percutaneous drilling and curettage or open curettage of the growth plate with radiographic control. Recurrent deformity is a rare but serious complication, and the surgeon should seek to fully ablate the physis.

In proximal femoral focal deficiency, arthrodesis of the knee results in improved function by bringing the extremity closer to the weight-bearing axis. Usually the distal femoral epiphysis is removed to shorten the residual limb so that there will be room in a prosthesis for a knee component.

The current approach to congenital vertical talus is to first perform serial casting to reduce the eversion and dorsiflexion of the forefoot. If the navicular is not fully reduced on the talus by casting, an open reduction of the talo-navicular joint can be done through a relatively small incision. The Achilles tendon is lengthened, as well as the toe extensors when necessary.

Knee disarticulation is a very functional level in children in that it allows end weight-bearing. Children are able to participate in athletics often using a prosthesis without a knee articulation. Frequently a distal femoral epiphyseodesis is needed to allow room for the prosthetic knee.

Procedure 43 Quadricepsplasty for Recurrent Dislocation of the Patella (Green Procedure)

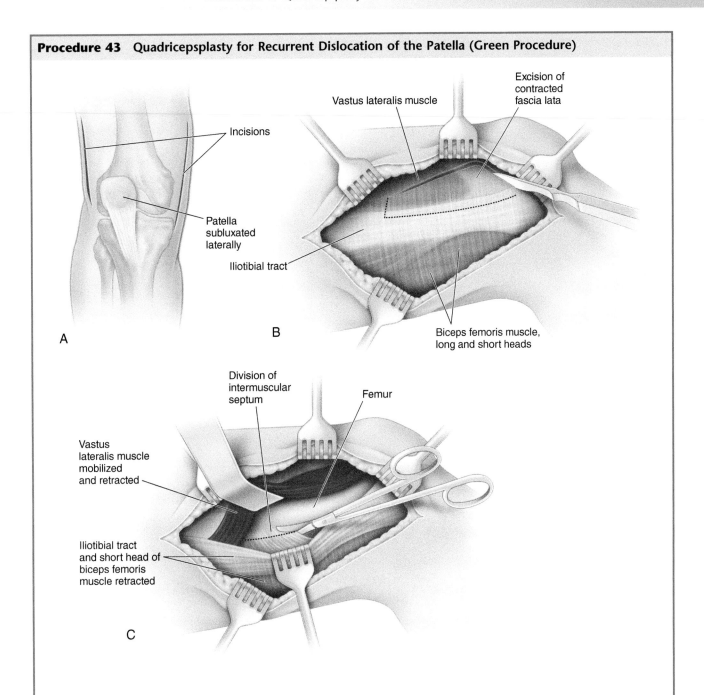

Operative Technique

A, The surgical approach is through two longitudinal skin incisions. The first incision is medial, beginning 3 cm medial and 4 cm proximal to the superior pole of the patella and extending distally to terminate at a point 2 cm distal and 1 cm medial to the proximal tibial tubercle. The lateral longitudinal skin incision begins at the joint line 2 cm lateral to the lateral margin of the patellar tendon and extends proximally for a distance of 1 to 10 cm. In this drawing, a J-shaped incision is illustrated; we do not recommend its use because the operative scar is ugly. The subcutaneous tissue and superficial fascia are divided, and the skin flaps are developed medially and laterally to expose the quadriceps muscle, patella, patellar tendon, patellar retinaculum, joint capsule, and iliotibial band.

B and **C,** Starting at a level 4 cm proximal to the lateral femoral condyle, a 7.5-cm segment of the fascia lata and the lateral intermuscular septum is excised. Next, abnormal attachments of the iliotibial band are divided, and the vastus lateralis muscle is widely mobilized from the deep surface of the fascia lata and its origin from the femur to allow free medial displacement of the patella. During this procedure, several muscular branches of the perforating arteries may be encountered, requiring coagulation or ligation.

Continued on following page

Procedure 43   Quadricepsplasty for Recurrent Dislocation of the Patella (Green Procedure), cont'd

D and **E,** The contracted iliotibial tract, patellar retinaculum, and lateral joint capsule are then longitudinally divided in their posterolateral portion to allow medial displacement of the patella. The lax medial joint capsule and patellar retinaculum are longitudinally incised, to be reefed later. The insertion of the vastus medialis, with its tendinous fibers and the periosteum of the patella, is detached from the medial and superior border of the patella by U-shaped incisions in the superoanterior and posteroinferior margins of the muscle. The synovial membrane is not incised unless inspection of the interior of the joint for loose bodies or chondromalacia of the patella is indicated. Next, the patella is displaced medially and the medial joint capsule is imbricated and tightly closed by reefing sutures. With the knee in complete extension, the medial patellar retinaculum is also imbricated by reefing sutures.

F, The superficial surface of the anterolateral third of the inferior half of the patella is then roughened with curved osteotomes and a curet. The vastus medialis tendon is transferred laterally and distally deep to the patellar bursa and sutured to the lateral border of the patellar tendon. The wounds are closed in layers and a well-molded cylinder cast is applied with the knee in neutral position or in 5 degrees of flexion.

Postoperative Care

Immobilization in the solid cast is continued for a period of 3 to 4 weeks. During this time the patient is permitted to walk with crutches with a three-point partial weight-bearing gait. Quadriceps muscle strength is maintained by isometric exercises in the solid cast. Then the cast is removed, and knee motion and muscle strength are gradually developed by flexion-extension exercises. A knee orthosis that holds the patella in reduced anatomic position and the knee in neutral extension is worn during the day for 4 weeks. Protection with crutches is continued until there is fair strength of the quadriceps muscle and 90 degrees of knee flexion.

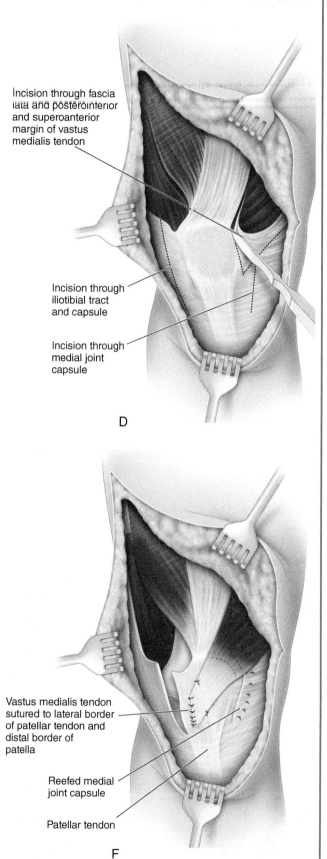

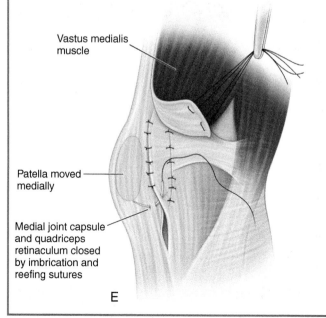

Procedure 44 Knee Fusion for Prosthetic Conversion in Proximal Focal Femoral Deficiency

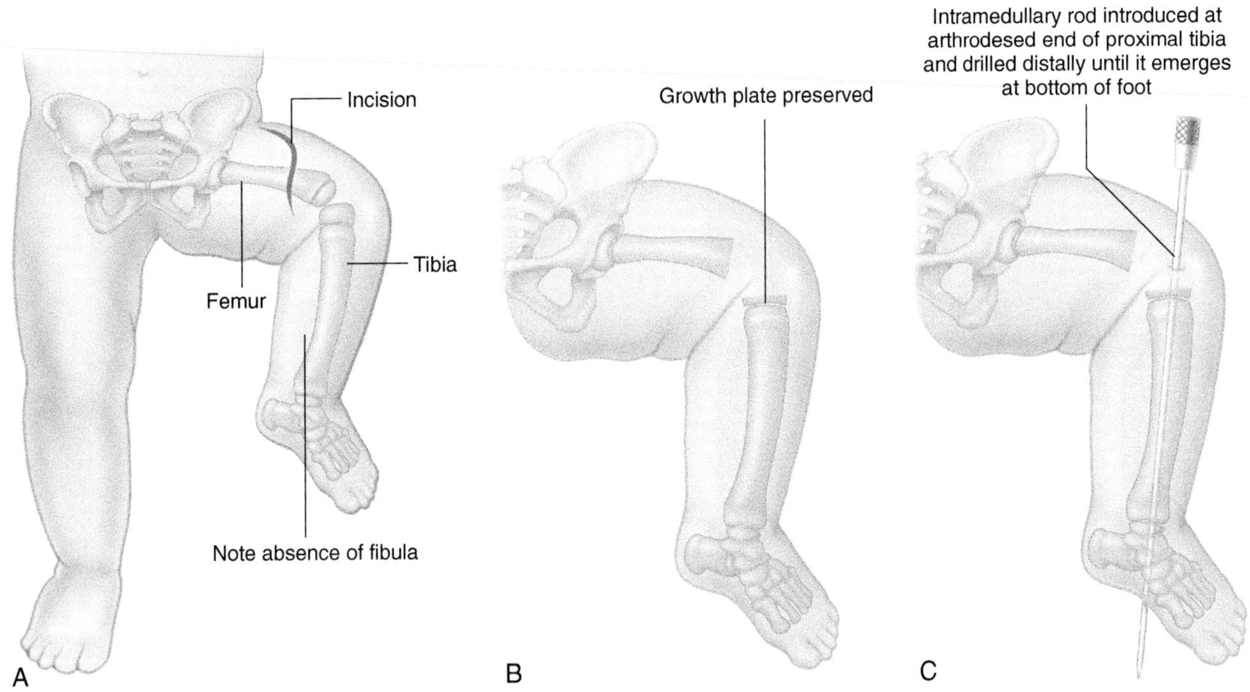

A

B

C

Arthrodesis of the knee converts the proximal focal femoral–deficient limb into a stable limb by removing the intercalated segment. The original technique included a Syme-type ankle disarticulation. Subsequent modifications offer the option of rotationplasty, which retains the foot.

Operative Technique

A, With the patient supine, an anterior S-shaped incision is made to expose the anterior aspect of the lower femur and upper tibia. Proximally, the incision is extended laterally to expose the lateral aspect of the upper femur.

B, The capsule and synovium of the knee joint are opened, and the articular cartilage of the upper end of the tibia is excised with an oscillating electric saw until the ossific nucleus of the epiphysis is seen. The distal femoral epiphysis is completely removed.

C, An 8-mm intramedullary nail is inserted. First it is inserted distally into the tibia, and it exits from the sole of the foot.

Continued on following page

Procedure 44   Knee Fusion for Prosthetic Conversion in Proximal Focal Femoral Deficiency, cont'd

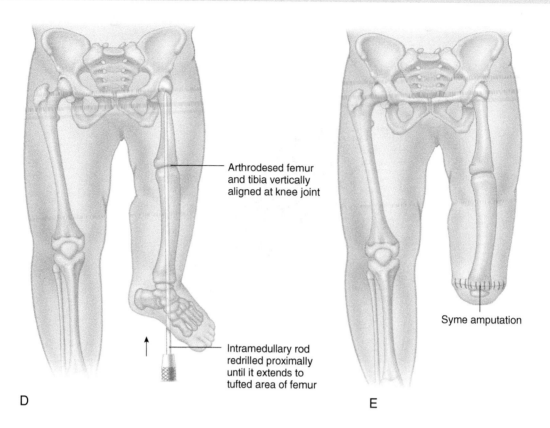

Arthrodesed femur
and tibia vertically
aligned at knee joint

Intramedullary rod
redrilled proximally
until it extends to
tufted area of femur

D

Syme amputation

E

D, The nail is then passed proximally into the femur, thus impacting the lower end of the femur and the upper epiphysis of the tibia in extension. Care is taken to provide proper rotational alignment of the lower limb and ensure that the fused knee is not in flexion. The intramedullary nail should be in the center of the physes of the distal femur and the proximal tibia to avoid growth retardation.

The wound is closed in routine fashion. A one-and-one-half spica cast is applied for immobilization.
E, Syme amputation may be performed at this time or later if desired. The intramedullary nail is removed after 6 weeks.

Procedure 45   Open Reduction of Dorsolateral Dislocation of the Talocalcaneonavicular Joint (Congenital Vertical Talus)

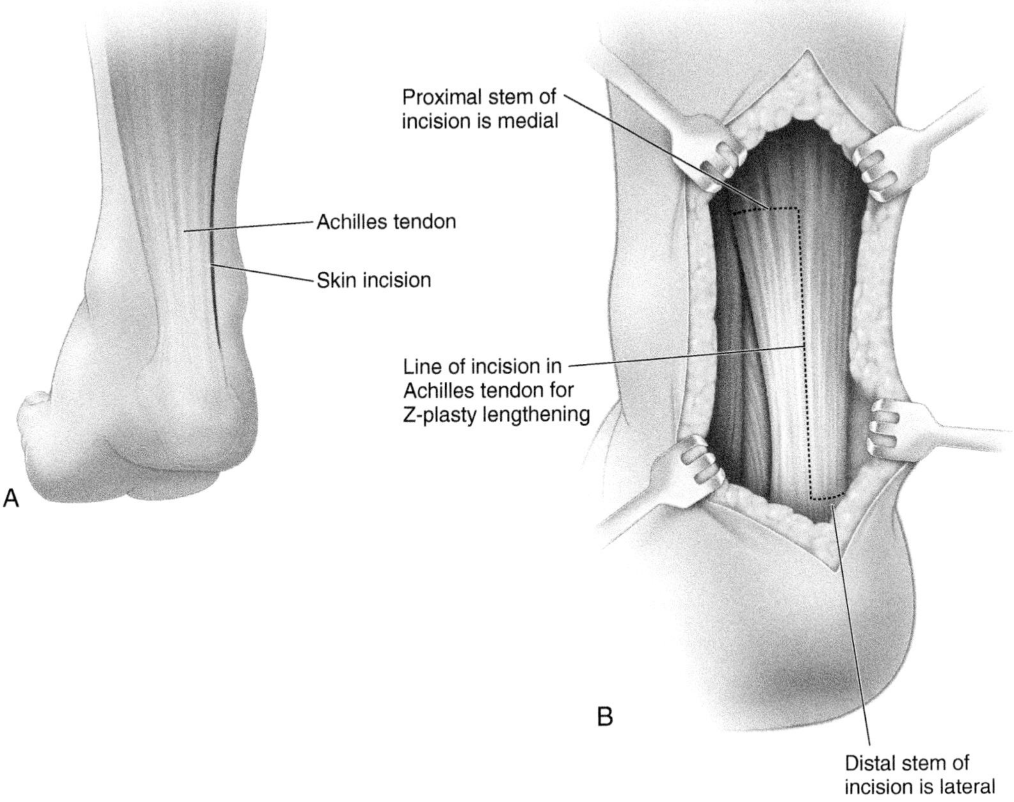

Proximal stem of incision is medial

Achilles tendon

Skin incision

Line of incision in Achilles tendon for Z-plasty lengthening

A

B

Distal stem of incision is lateral

Operative Technique

A, A longitudinal incision is made lateral to the tendo calcaneus, beginning at the heel and extending proximally for a distance of 7 to 10 cm. The subcutaneous tissue and tendon sheath are divided in line with the skin incision, and the wound flaps are retracted to expose the Achilles tendon.

B, Z-plasty lengthening is performed in the anteroposterior plane. With a knife, the Achilles tendon is divided longitudinally into lateral and medial halves for a distance of 5 to 7 cm. The distal end of the lateral half is detached from the calcaneus to prevent recurrence of valgus deformity of the heel; the medial half is divided proximally. When the equinus deformity is not marked, sliding lengthening of the heel cord is performed.

Continued on following page

Procedure 45   Open Reduction of Dorsolateral Dislocation of the Talocalcaneonavicular Joint (Congenital Vertical Talus), cont'd

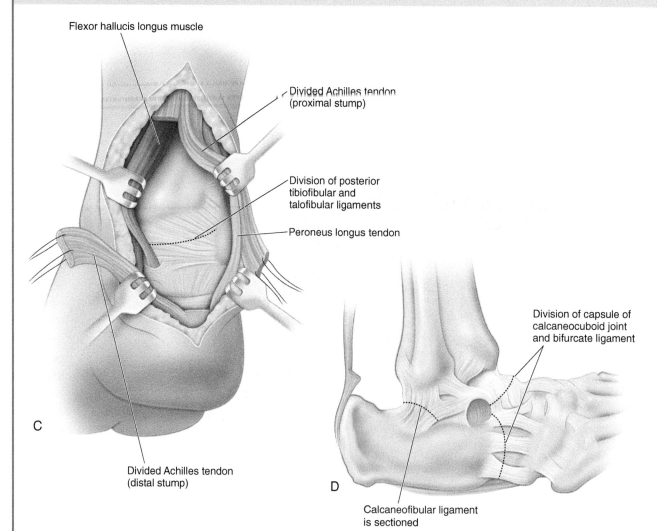

Flexor hallucis longus muscle

Divided Achilles tendon (proximal stump)

Division of posterior tibiofibular and talofibular ligaments

Peroneus longus tendon

C

Divided Achilles tendon (distal stump)

Division of capsule of calcaneocuboid joint and bifurcate ligament

D

Calcaneofibular ligament is sectioned

C and D, A posterior capsulotomy of the ankle and subtalar joint is performed if necessary. The calcaneofibular ligament is sectioned. The thickened capsule of the calcaneocuboid joint and the bifurcate ligament are divided through a separate lateral incision. The Cincinnati transverse incision is an alternative surgical approach; it is preferred by these authors. E, The incision is a modified Cincinnati incision that passes beneath the medial malleolus just past the Achilles tendon posteriorly and proceeds dorsally over the navicular just past the extensor tendons.

F and G, The posterior tibial tendon is identified, dissected, and divided at its insertion to the tuberosity of the navicular. The end of the tendon is marked with 0 Mersilene suture for later reattachment. The articular surface of the head of the talus points steeply downward and medially to the sole of the foot and is covered by the capsule and ligament. The navicular will be found against the dorsal aspect of the neck of the talus, where it locks the talus in a vertical position. The pathologic anatomy of the ligaments and capsule is noted, and the incisions are planned so that a secure capsuloplasty can be performed and the talus maintained in its normal anatomic position. Circulation to the talus is another

important consideration; it should be disturbed as little as possible by exercising great care and gentleness during dissection. Avascular necrosis of the talus is always a potential serious complication of open reduction. The plantar calcaneonavicular ligament is identified and divided distally from its attachment to the sustentaculum tali, and 00 Mersilene suture is inserted in its end for later reattachment. The talonavicular articulation is exposed by a T incision. The transverse limb of the T is made distally over the tibionavicular ligament (the anterior portion of the deltoid ligament) and over the dorsal and medial portions of the talonavicular ligament. A cuff of capsule is kept attached to the navicular for plication on completion of surgery. The longitudinal limb of the incision is made over the head and neck of the talus inferiorly.

The articular surface of the head of the talus is identified, and a large threaded Kirschner wire is inserted in its center. With a skid and the leverage of the Kirschner wire, the head and neck of the talus are lifted dorsally and the forefoot is manipulated into plantar flexion and inversion to bring the articular surfaces of the navicular and head of the talus into normal anatomic position.

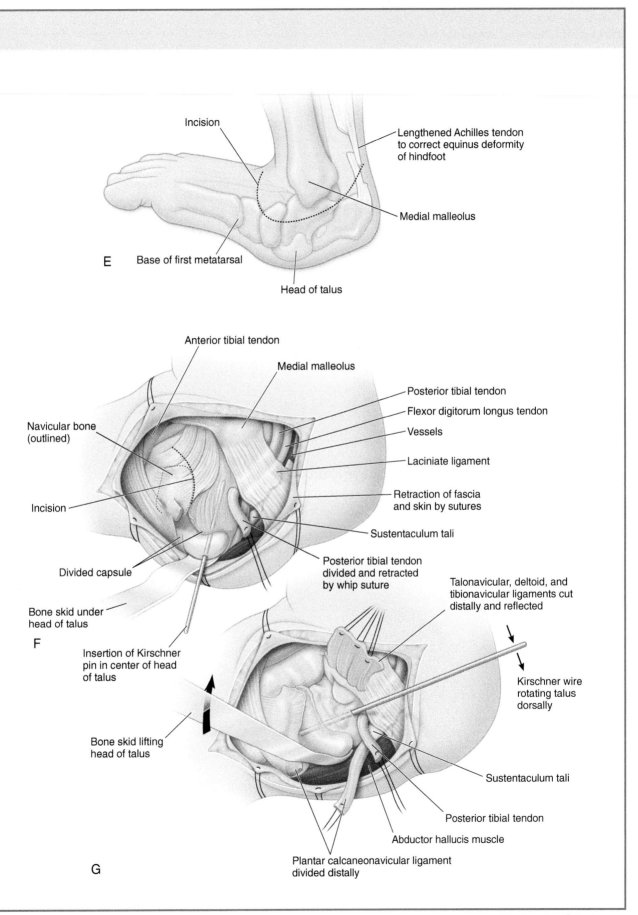

Incision

Lengthened Achilles tendon
to correct equinus deformity
of hindfoot

Medial malleolus

E   Base of first metatarsal

Head of talus

Anterior tibial tendon

Medial malleolus

Posterior tibial tendon

Flexor digitorum longus tendon

Navicular bone
(outlined)

Vessels

Laciniate ligament

Retraction of fascia
and skin by sutures

Incision

Sustentaculum tali

Posterior tibial tendon
divided and retracted
by whip suture

Divided capsule

Talonavicular, deltoid, and
tibionavicular ligaments cut
distally and reflected

Bone skid under
head of talus

F

Insertion of Kirschner
pin in center of head
of talus

Kirschner wire
rotating talus
dorsally

Bone skid lifting
head of talus

Sustentaculum tali

Posterior tibial tendon

Abductor hallucis muscle

G

Plantar calcaneonavicular ligament
divided distally

Continued on following page

Procedure 45   Open Reduction of Dorsolateral Dislocation of the Talocalcaneonavicular Joint (Congenital Vertical Talus), cont'd

H, The Kirschner wire is drilled retrograde into the navicular, cuneiform, and first metatarsal bones to maintain the reduction. Radiographs of the foot are obtained at this time to verify the reduction.

In severe cases, the calcaneocuboid and talocalcaneal interosseous ligaments may prevent reduction of the laterally subluxated Chopart and subtalar joints. They are divided when necessary to allow reduction. In addition, the extensor hallucis, extensor digitorum longus, and occasionally the peroneals may be contracted. They should be Z-lengthened to allow reduction of the foot into plantar flexion. These releases require extension of the incision over the dorsum of the foot.

I and J, A careful capsuloplasty is very important for maintaining the reduction and normal anatomic relationship of the talus and navicular. The redundant inferior part of the capsule should be tightened by plication and overlapping of its free edges. First, the plantar-proximal segment of the T of the capsule is pulled dorsally and distally and sutured to the dorsal corner of the inner surface of the distal capsule. Next, the dorsoproximal segment of the T is brought plantarward and distally over the plantar-proximal segment of the capsule and sutured to the plantar corner on the inner surface of the distal capsule. Interrupted sutures are then used to tighten the capsule on its plantar and medial aspects by bringing the distal segment over the proximal segments.

The plantar calcaneonavicular ligament is sutured under tension to the base of the first metatarsal. To tighten the posterior tibial tendon under the head of the talus, it is advanced distally and sutured to the inferior surface of the first cuneiform.

The anterior tibial tendon may be transferred to provide additional dynamic force for maintaining the navicular in correct relation to the talus. The tendon is detached from its insertion to the medial cuneiform and first metatarsal bone, and dissected free proximally and medially for a distance of 5 cm. It is then redirected to pass along the medial aspect of the neck of the talus and beneath the head of the talus, where it is fixed to the inferior aspects of the talus and navicular with 00 Mersilene sutures. Normally, the lower end of the anterior tibial tendon may be split near its insertion. Often the authors leave the attachment to the first metatarsal intact and divide only the insertion to the medial cuneiform. The tendon is split (if not normally bifurcated), and the portion to the medial cuneiform bone is transferred to the head of the talus and the navicular. Sometimes, after adequate capsuloplasty, the reduction of the talonavicular joint is so stable that anterior tibial transfer is not necessary to restore support to the head of the talus.

K, The wounds are then closed in routine fashion. The Kirschner wire across the talonavicular joint is cut subcutaneously. To maintain the normal anatomic relationship of the os calcis to the talus, a Kirschner wire is inserted transversely in the os calcis and incorporated into the cast. An alternative method is to pass the wire from the sole of the foot upward through the calcaneus into the talus. The authors prefer the former because it controls the heel in the cast and prevents recurrence of both equinus deformity and eversion of the hindfoot. An above-knee cast is applied with the knee in 45 degrees of flexion, the ankle in 10 to 15 degrees of dorsiflexion, the heel in 10 degrees of inversion, and the forefoot in plantar flexion and inversion. The longitudinal arch and the heel in the cast are well molded.

Postoperative Care

The Kirschner wires are removed after 6 weeks. The foot is placed in a walking cast for another 4 to 6 weeks to maintain correction. Further splinting is necessary only in children with neurologic abnormalities or those with arthrogryposis.

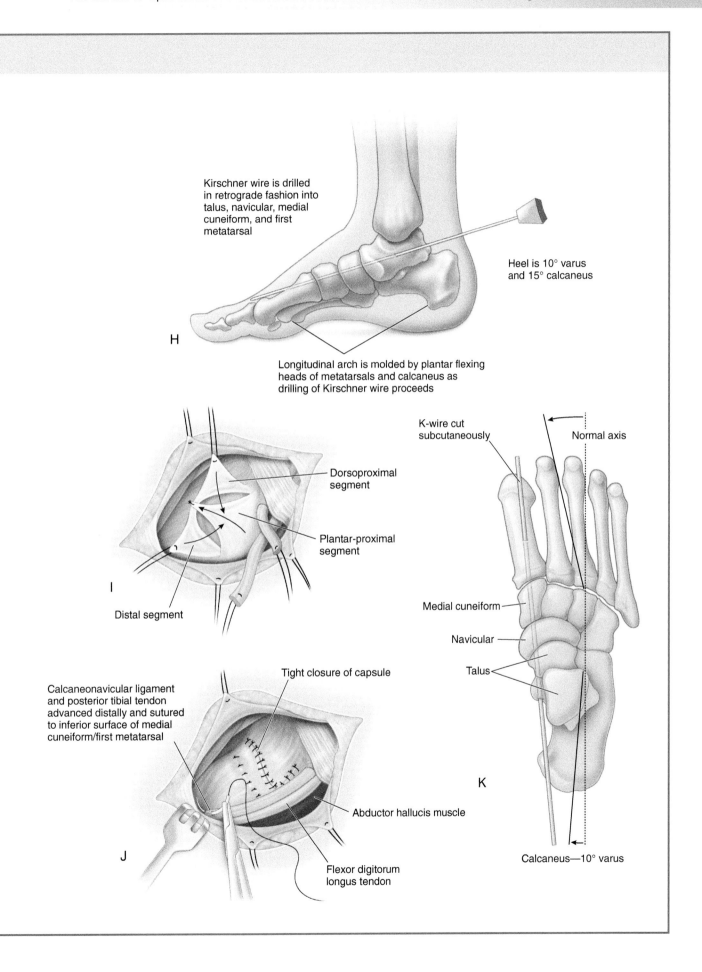

Kirschner wire is drilled in retrograde fashion into talus, navicular, medial cuneiform, and first metatarsal

Heel is 10° varus and 15° calcaneus

Longitudinal arch is molded by plantar flexing heads of metatarsals and calcaneus as drilling of Kirschner wire proceeds

H

Dorsoproximal segment

Plantar-proximal segment

Distal segment

I

K-wire cut subcutaneously

Normal axis

Medial cuneiform

Navicular

Talus

K

Calcaneonavicular ligament and posterior tibial tendon advanced distally and sutured to inferior surface of medial cuneiform/first metatarsal

Tight closure of capsule

Abductor hallucis muscle

Flexor digitorum longus tendon

J

Calcaneus—10° varus

Procedure 46 Plantar Fasciotomy

A, A 1- to 2-cm incision is made over the medial aspect of the plantar fascia, which is easily palpable in the sole of the foot.
B, The plantar fascia can be seen within the wound.

C, The fascia is isolated on its dorsal and plantar surfaces, thus protecting the plantar divisions of the tibial nerve. The fascia is then divided with scissors across the sole of the foot.

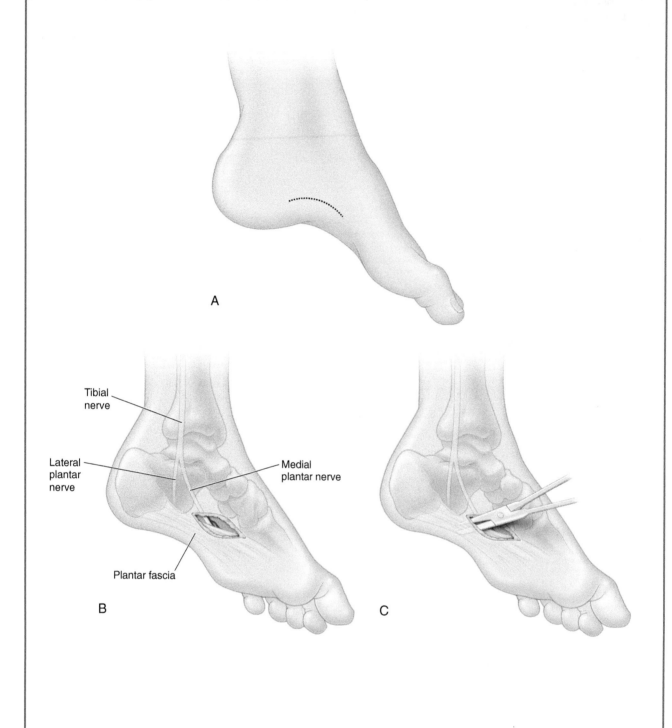

A

Tibial
nerve

Lateral
plantar
nerve

Medial
plantar nerve

Plantar fascia

B

C

Procedure 47 Transfer of the Long Toe Extensors to the Heads of the Metatarsals (Jones Transfer)

A, A longitudinal incision is made on the dorsomedial aspect of the first metatarsal from the base of the proximal phalanx to the proximal fourth of the metatarsal shaft. The incision should be placed medial to the extensor hallucis longus tendon, toward the second metatarsal. The subcutaneous tissue is divided and the wound flaps retracted with 0 silk sutures. The digital nerves and vessels should not be injured.

B, The extensor hallucis longus and brevis tendons are identified and sectioned at the base of the proximal phalanx. An alternative technique is to leave the insertion of the extensor hallucis brevis tendon intact; the stump of the extensor hallucis longus tendon is sutured to the intact brevis tendon.

C, Silk whip sutures (00) are inserted into the ends of the long and short toe extensors. The long toe extensor is dissected free and its sheath is thoroughly excised with a sharp scalpel as far proximally as possible.

D, The epiphyseal plate of the first metatarsal is proximal, whereas that of the lateral four metatarsals is distal in location. The extensor hallucis longus tendon is transferred to the head of the first metatarsal. The long toe extensors of the lesser toes are transferred to the distal third of the metatarsal shafts, with care taken to not disturb the growth plate. When the patient is older than 10 to 12 years, the tendons are transferred to the heads of the metatarsals because by then growth of the foot is almost complete.

With small Chandler elevator retractors, the soft tissues are retracted. The periosteum is not stripped. Through a stab wound in the periosteum, a hole is drilled in the center of the first metatarsal head and enlarged to receive the tendon. The extensor hallucis longus tendon is passed through the hole in the first metatarsal in a medial-to-lateral direction and sutured to itself with the forefoot in maximal dorsiflexion.

E, The extensor hallucis brevis tendon is then sutured to the stump of the long toe extensor while holding the toe in neutral extension or in 10 degrees of dorsiflexion.

A similar technique is used to transfer the long extensor tendons of the lesser toes. Longitudinal incisions are made between the second and third metatarsals and between the fourth and fifth metatarsals. The extensor brevis tendon of the little toe is either absent or not of adequate size to transfer to the stump of the longus.

The tourniquet is released, and complete hemostasis is obtained. The wounds are closed with interrupted sutures.

Postoperative Care

A cast with a sturdy, well-padded toe plate is applied and worn for 4 to 6 weeks. The plantar aspect of the metatarsals should be well padded to prevent ulceration. Special muscle training for the transferred tendons is not required because this is an in-phase transfer.

Continued on following page

Procedure 47   Transfer of the Long Toe Extensors to the Heads of the Metatarsals (Jones Transfer), cont'd

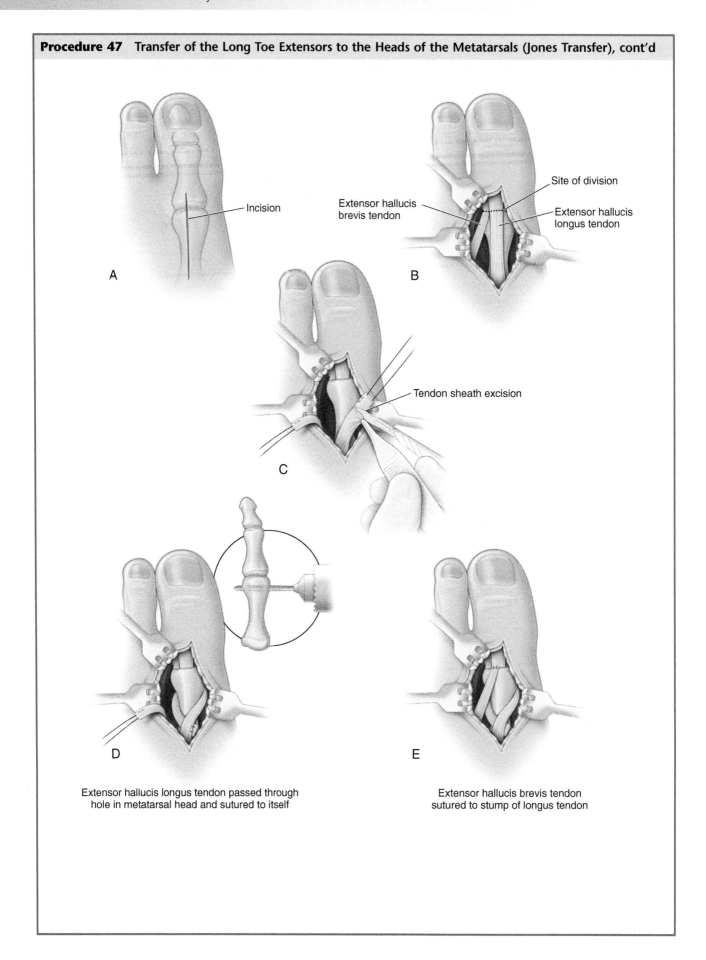

A — Incision

B — Extensor hallucis brevis tendon / Site of division / Extensor hallucis longus tendon

C — Tendon sheath excision

D — Extensor hallucis longus tendon passed through hole in metatarsal head and sutured to itself

E — Extensor hallucis brevis tendon sutured to stump of longus tendon

Procedure 48 **Dwyer Lateral Wedge Resection of the Calcaneus for Pes Cavus** (see Video 8)

The forefoot equinus deformity is corrected first, either by plantar soft tissue release or by dorsal wedge tarsal resection, depending on the age of the patient and the severity of the deformity. Closing lateral wedge resection of the os calcis is designed to correct a varus deformity of a hindfoot in which the heel is of adequate height and size.

Operative Technique

A, A 5-cm long oblique incision is made on the lateral aspect of the calcaneus parallel to but 1.5 cm posterior and inferior to the peroneus longus tendon. The subcutaneous tissue is divided and the wound flaps are retracted. **B and C,** The peroneal tendons are identified and retracted dorsally and distally. The calcaneofibular ligament is sectioned, and the periosteum is incised. The lateral surface of the calcaneus is subperiosteally exposed; with Chandler elevator retractors, the superior and inferior aspects of the calcaneus are partially exposed. With a pair of osteotomes of adequate width, a wedge of the os calcis with its base directed laterally is excised. The site of osteotomy is immediately inferior and posterior to the peroneus longus tendon. The medial cortex should be left intact. The width of the base of the wedge depends on the severity of the varus deformity of the heel.

D, Next, a Steinmann pin is inserted transversely across the posterior segment of the calcaneus. The forefoot is dorsiflexed to put tension on the Achilles tendon, and with the Steinmann pin serving as a lever, the bone gap is closed. The heel should be in 5 degrees of valgus. The wound is closed and an above-knee cast is applied, the pin being incorporated in the cast. The knee is in 45 degrees of flexion.

Postoperative Care

The cast, pin, and sutures are removed in 4 weeks. A below-knee walking cast is then applied for an additional 2 weeks, by which time the osteotomy should be healed.

Continued on following page

Procedure 48   Dwyer Lateral Wedge Resection of the Calcaneus for Pes Cavus, cont'd

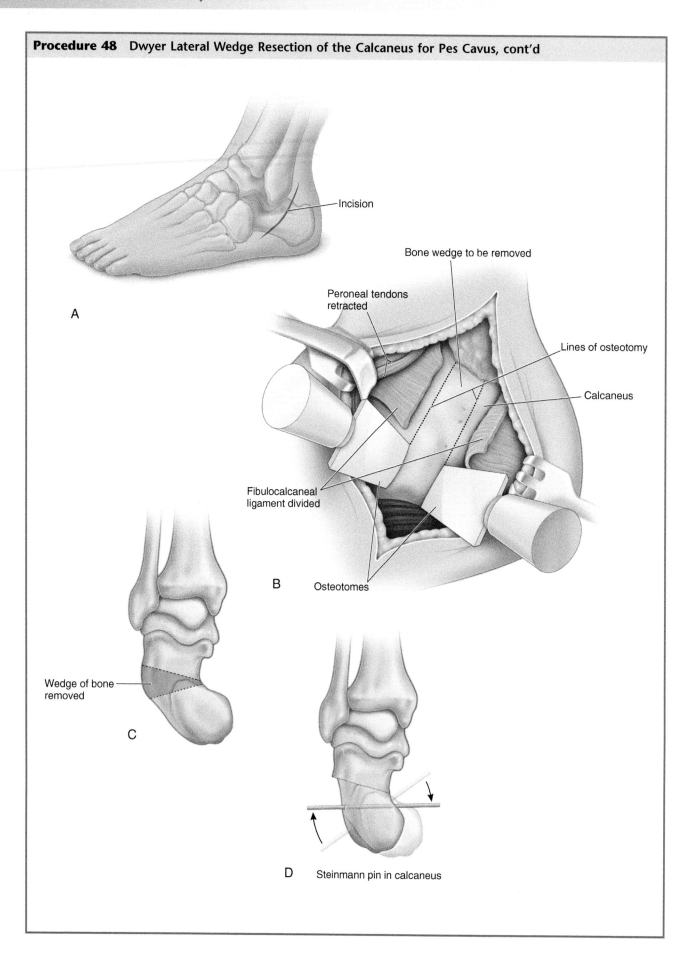

A

Incision

Bone wedge to be removed

Peroneal tendons
retracted

Lines of osteotomy

Calcaneus

Fibulocalcaneal
ligament divided

B   Osteotomes

Wedge of bone
removed

C

D   Steinmann pin in calcaneus

Procedure 49   Dorsal Wedge Resection for Pes Cavus

The dorsal aspect of the tarsal bones may be exposed by several means. Cole and Japas make a single dorsal longitudinal incision approximately 6 to 8 cm long in the midline of the foot and centered over the midtarsal arch (naviculocuneiform junction). Subcutaneous tissue is divided, and the long toe extensors are identified and separated. The plane between the long extensor tendons of the second and third toes is developed, and the extensor digitorum brevis muscle is identified, elevated, and retracted laterally with the peroneus brevis tendon. The anterior tibial tendon and the long extensor tendons of the second and big toes are retracted medially. The periosteum is incised, longitudinally elevated, and retracted medially and laterally.[15,35] Meary makes two longitudinal incisions, each approximately 5 to 6 cm in length, on the dorsum of the foot. The medial incision is parallel to the longitudinal axis of the second metatarsal and is centered over the intermediate cuneiform bone. The extensor hallucis longus tendon, dorsalis pedis vessels, and anterior tibial tendon are identified, dissected free, and retracted medially. The lateral incision is approximately 3 cm long and is centered over the cuboid bone. The peroneus brevis is identified and retracted laterally.

We use two longitudinal incisions, one dorsolateral and the other medial.

Operative Technique

A and **B,** Two longitudinal skin incisions are made. The medial incision, approximately 5 cm long, is made over the medial aspect of the navicular and first cuneiform bones in the interval between the anterior tibial and posterior tibial tendons. The subcutaneous tissue is divided. The anterior tibial tendon is retracted dorsally; the posterior tibial tendon is partially detached from the tuberosity of the navicular and retracted plantarward to expose the medial and dorsal aspects of the navicular and first cuneiform bones. The dorsolateral incision, approximately 4 cm long, is centered over the cuboid bone. The extensor brevis muscle is identified, elevated, and retracted distally

and laterally with the peroneus brevis tendon. The long toe extensors are retracted medially.

C, Next, through the medial wound, the capsule and periosteum of the navicular and first cuneiform bones are incised and elevated. The soft tissues are retracted dorsally and plantarward with Chandler elevator retractors. The capsule of the talonavicular joint should not be disturbed. If in doubt, the surgeon should obtain radiographs to identify the tarsal bones with certainty.

D and **E,** With osteotomes, a wedge of bone is excised, including the naviculocuneiform articulation. The base of the wedge is dorsal, its width depends on the severity of the forefoot equinus deformity to be corrected. The wedge osteotomy of the cuboid is completed through the dorsolateral incision.

F, The forefoot is then manipulated into dorsiflexion. If the plantar fascia is contracted, a plantar fasciotomy is performed. In severe cases the short plantar muscles are also sectioned. The first cuneiform bone should be dorsally displaced over the navicular bone. Two Steinmann pins are inserted to transfix the tarsal osteotomy. The medial pin is inserted into the shaft of the first metatarsal and directed posteriorly through the first cuneiform, across the osteotomy site, and into the navicular and head of the talus. The lateral pin is started posteriorly along the longitudinal axis of the calcaneus and directed across the calcaneocuboid joint and into the cuboid and base of the fifth metatarsal. (Meary uses staples to maintain the position of the osteotomy.) Radiographs are obtained to verify the position of the pins and maintenance of correction of the forefoot equinus deformity. The tourniquet is released, and complete hemostasis is obtained. The incisions are closed. The pins are cut subcutaneously, and a below-knee cast is applied.

Postoperative Care

The foot and leg are immobilized for 6 weeks, at which time the cast, pins, and sutures are removed. A new below-knee walking cast is applied and worn for another 2 to 4 weeks.

Continued on following page

Procedure 49   Dorsal Wedge Resection for Pes Cavus, cont'd

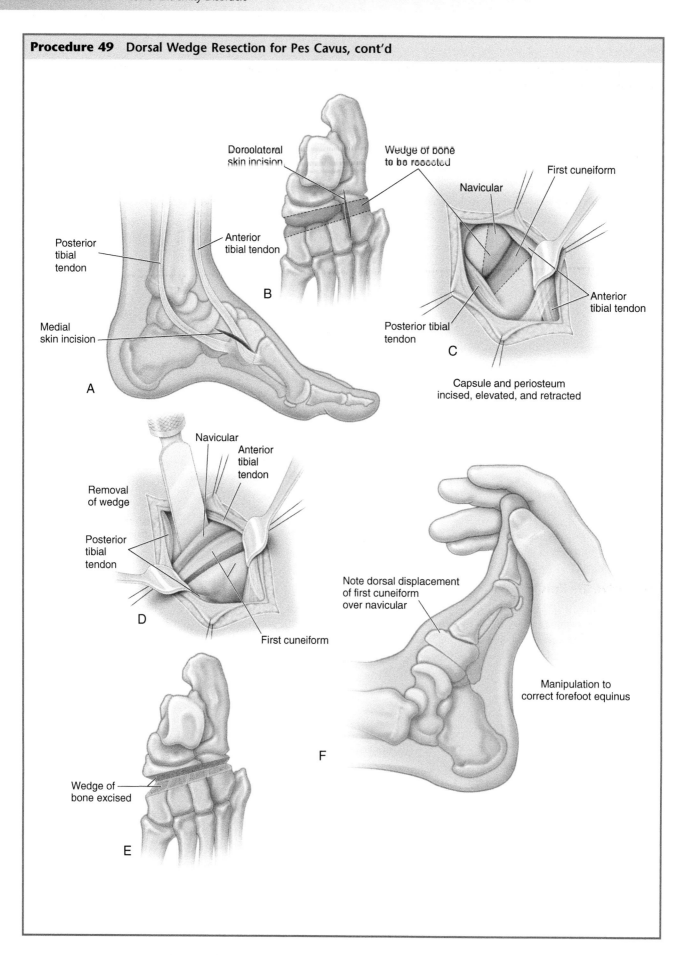

Posterior tibial tendon

Medial skin incision

A

Dorsolateral skin incision

Wedge of bone to be resected

Anterior tibial tendon

B

Navicular

First cuneiform

Posterior tibial tendon

Anterior tibial tendon

Capsule and periosteum incised, elevated, and retracted

C

Removal of wedge

Navicular

Anterior tibial tendon

Posterior tibial tendon

First cuneiform

D

Wedge of bone excised

E

Note dorsal displacement of first cuneiform over navicular

Manipulation to correct forefoot equinus

F

Procedure 50   Japas V-Osteotomy of the Tarsus

Operative Technique

A, The dorsal aspect of the tarsal bones is exposed through a longitudinal incision 6 to 8 cm long in the midline of the foot (i.e., between the second and third rays) and centered over the midtarsal area at the naviculocuneiform junction.

B and C, The subcutaneous tissue is divided. The superficial nerves are isolated and protected. The long toe extensor tendons are identified and separated, and the plane between those of the second and third toes is developed. The extensor digitorum brevis muscle is identified, elevated extraperiosteally, and retracted laterally with the peroneal tendons. The extensor hallucis longus tendon, dorsalis pedis vessels, and anterior tibial tendon are identified, dissected free, and retracted medially. The osteotomy site is exposed extraperiosteally.

The talonavicular joint is identified next. Caution! Do not injure the midtarsal joint and compromise its function. If bony landmarks are distorted, radiographs are obtained for proper orientation. Inadvertent partial ostectomy of the head of the talus will result in aseptic necrosis and traumatic arthritis. The V line of the osteotomy is marked. Its apex is in the midline of the foot at the height of the arch of the cavus deformity, its medial limb extends to the middle of the medial cuneiform and exits proximal to the cuneiform–first metatarsal joint, and its lateral limb extends to the middle of the cuboid and emerges proximal to the cuboid–fifth metatarsal joint. Often the V is shallow, shaped more like a dome.

Continued on following page

Procedure 50   Japas V-Osteotomy of the Tarsus, cont'd

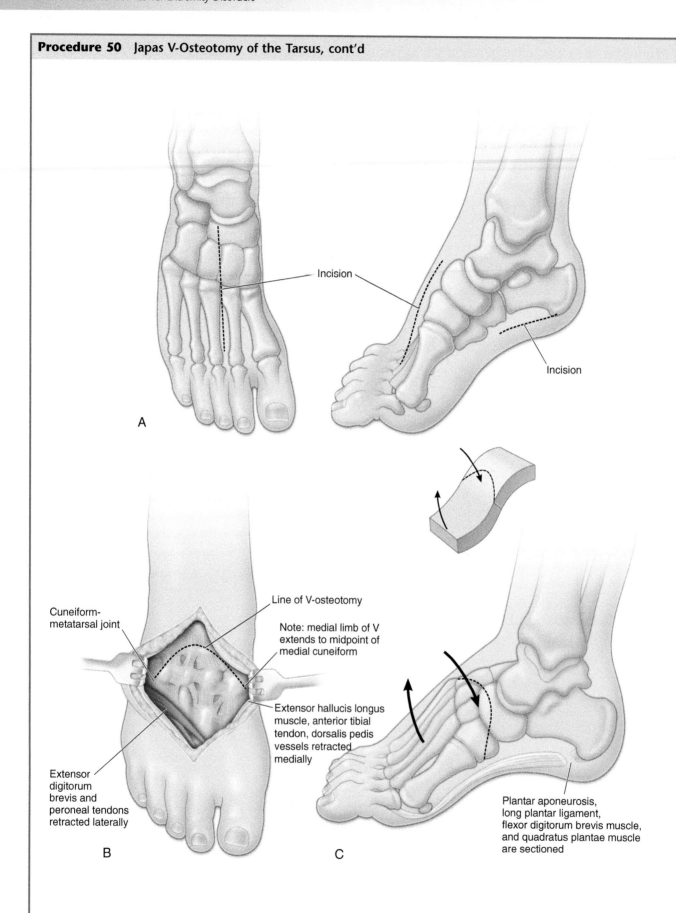

Incision

Incision

A

Line of V-osteotomy

Note: medial limb of V
extends to midpoint of
medial cuneiform

Cuneiform-
metatarsal joint

Extensor hallucis longus
muscle, anterior tibial
tendon, dorsalis pedis
vessels retracted
medially

Extensor
digitorum
brevis and
peroneal tendons
retracted laterally

Plantar aponeurosis,
long plantar ligament,
flexor digitorum brevis muscle,
and quadratus plantae muscle
are sectioned

B

C

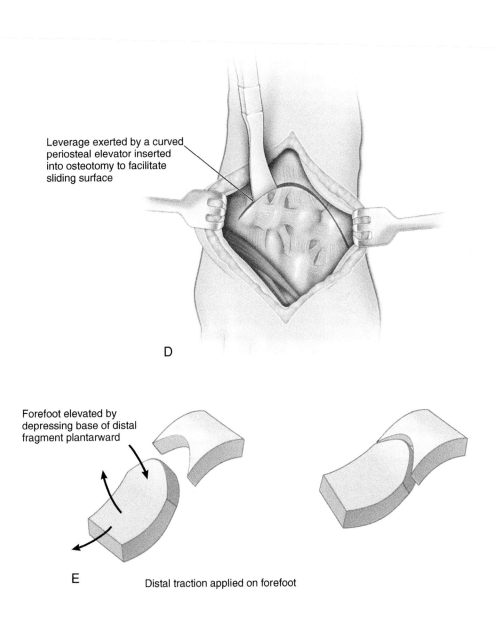

Leverage exerted by a curved periosteal elevator inserted into osteotomy to facilitate sliding surface

D

Forefoot elevated by depressing base of distal fragment plantarward

E   Distal traction applied on forefoot

D and **E,** The osteotomy is begun with an oscillating bone saw and completed with an osteotome. Splintering of the ends of the medial and lateral limbs should be avoided. Next, a curved periosteal elevator is inserted into the osteotomy site, manual traction is applied on the forefoot, and with the elevator used as a lever, the base of the distal fragment is depressed plantarward. This maneuver corrects the cavus deformity and lengthens the concave plantar surface of the foot. The foot is not shortened as it would be by resection of a bone wedge, and any abduction or adduction deformity can be corrected if necessary.

Continued on following page

Procedure 50 Japas V-Osteotomy of the Tarsus, cont'd

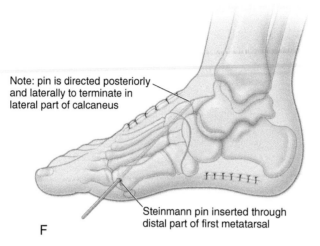

Note: pin is directed posteriorly and laterally to terminate in lateral part of calcaneus

Steinmann pin inserted through distal part of first metatarsal

F

F, Once the desired alignment is achieved, a single Steinmann pin is inserted through the distal part of the first metatarsal and directed posteriorly and laterally to terminate in the lateral part of the calcaneus or the cuboid. Radiographs are obtained to verify the completeness of correction. The tourniquet is then removed, hemostasis is achieved, and the wound is closed with interrupted sutures. The pin is cut subcutaneously, and a below-knee cast is applied.

Procedure 51 Correction of Hammer Toe by Resection and Arthrodesis of the Proximal Interphalangeal Joint

Operative Technique

A, A 3- to 4-cm longitudinal incision is made over the dorsal aspect of the proximal interphalangeal (PIP) joint parallel to and at the lateral border of the extensor digitorum longus tendon. The subcutaneous tissue is divided and the skin flaps are retracted.

B, The long extensor tendon is split and retracted to expose the capsule of the PIP joint. The digital vessels and nerves are protected from injury. A transverse incision is made in the capsule, and the joint surfaces are widely exposed.

C and **D,** With a rongeur, wedges of bone based dorsally are resected from the head of the proximal phalanx and the base of the middle phalanx. Enough bone should be removed to allow correction of the deformity.

E and **F,** The proximal and middle phalanges are held together by internal fixation with a Kirschner wire that is inserted retrogradely. The Kirschner wire should not cross the metatarsophalangeal joint. The cancellous bony surfaces of the middle and proximal phalanges should be apposed, and the rotational alignment should be correct. The capsule is resutured tightly by reefing. The wound is closed in a routine manner. The end of the Kirschner wire is bent 90 degrees and cut, with 0.5 cm of wire left protruding through the skin.

Postoperative Care

A below-knee walking cast is applied with a band of casting material protecting the toe. The wire and cast are removed in 6 weeks, when radiographs show fusion of the interphalangeal joint.

Continued on following page

Procedure 51 **Correction of Hammer Toe by Resection and Arthrodesis of the Proximal Interphalangeal Joint, cont'd**

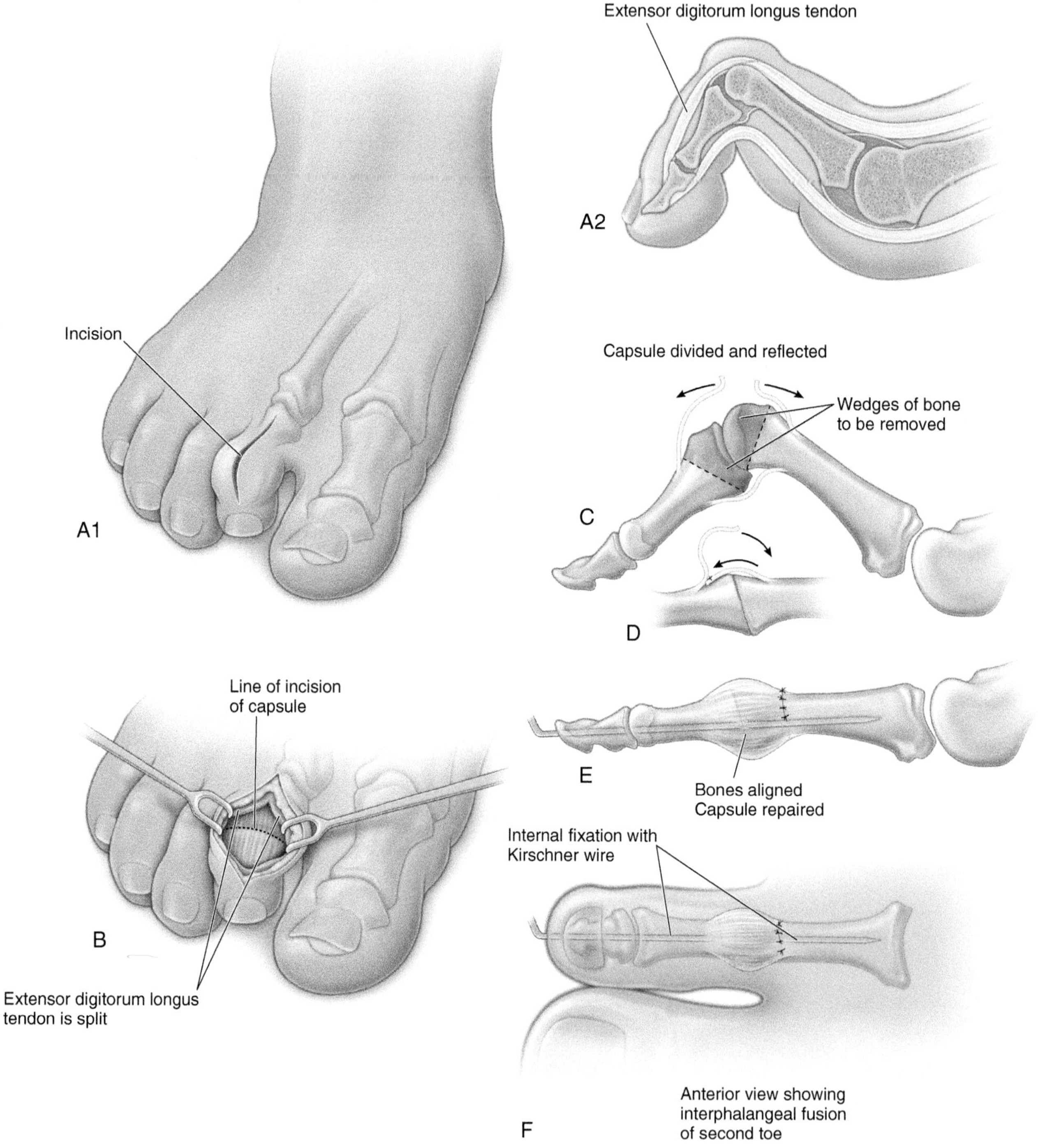

Extensor digitorum longus tendon

A2

Incision

A1

Capsule divided and reflected

Wedges of bone to be removed

C

D

Line of incision of capsule

B

Extensor digitorum longus tendon is split

E

Bones aligned
Capsule repaired

Internal fixation with Kirschner wire

F

Anterior view showing interphalangeal fusion of second toe

Procedure 52 Epiphysiodesis of the Distal Femur (the Green Modification of the Phemister Technique)

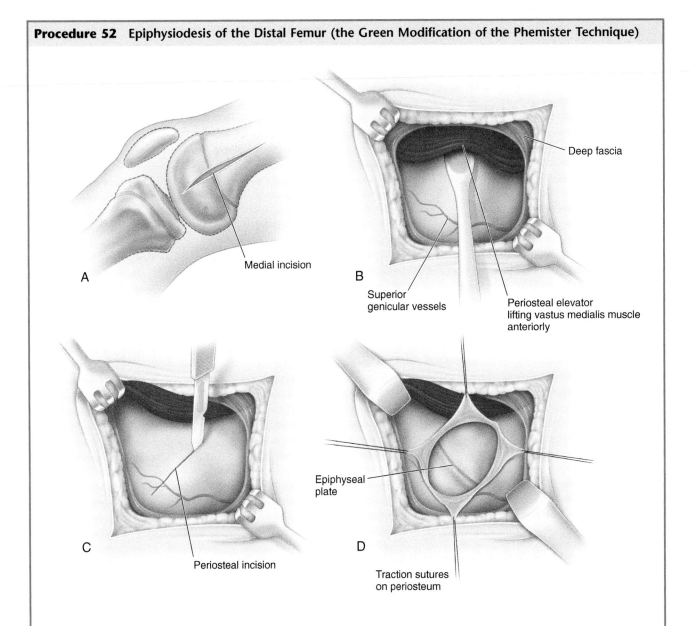

A, Medial incision

B, Deep fascia; Superior genicular vessels; Periosteal elevator lifting vastus medialis muscle anteriorly

C, Periosteal incision

D, Epiphyseal plate; Traction sutures on periosteum

Operative Technique

A, The knee is supported in 20 to 30 degrees of flexion, and the joint line is identified. First, the medial aspect of the distal femur is exposed. Beginning 1 cm superior to the joint line, a longitudinal incision approximately 3 cm long is made midway between the anterior and posterior margins of the femoral condyles. The subcutaneous tissue and deep fascia are divided in line with the skin incision.
B, Following the anterior surface of the medial intermuscular septum, the vastus medialis muscle is lifted anteriorly with a blunt periosteal elevator. The suprapatellar pouch should not be entered. In the inferior margin of the wound, the capsule and reflected synovial membrane of the knee joint are gently elevated and retracted with blunt instruments distally. The superior medial genicular vessels traverse the wound; it is best to coagulate them to prevent troublesome bleeding later.

C, A midline longitudinal incision is made in the periosteum, starting proximally and extending throughout the extent of the wound.
D, The medial distal femoral physis is exposed by raising anterior and posterior flaps of periosteum by subperiosteal dissection; it appears as a white, glistening transverse line that is softer than adjacent cancellous bone. Some surgeons prefer to make a longitudinal I-shaped incision in the periosteum to expose the growth plate. The periosteum is gently retracted. Rough traction and shredding of the periosteum should be avoided. If necessary, elevators are placed subperiosteally on the anterior and posterior aspects of the distal femur for adequate exposure. Dull right-angled retractors are used for proximal and distal retraction.

Continued on following page

Procedure 52   Epiphysiodesis of the Distal Femur (the Green Modification of the Phemister Technique), cont'd

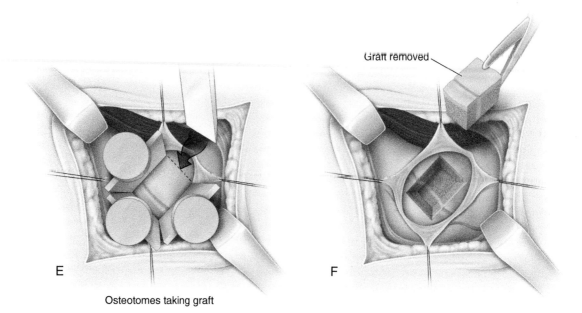

Osteotomes taking graft

E and F, With matched pairs of osteotomes, a rectangular piece of bone $1\frac{1}{8}$ to $1\frac{1}{2}$ inches long and $\frac{1}{2}$- to $\frac{5}{8}$-inch wide is excised. The epiphyseal plate should be at the junction of the distal one third and proximal two thirds of the length of bone graft resected, at a point equidistant between the anterior and posterior surfaces of the femur. The posterior cortex of the femur should not be broken. The depth of the bone graft is $\frac{1}{2}$ to $\frac{3}{4}$ inch. Because of the flare of the femoral condyles, the anterior and posterior osteotomes should be tilted somewhat distally so that they are perpendicular to the medial surface of the femur. Following removal of the osteotomes, the completeness of the osteotomy is checked with a thin ($\frac{3}{8}$- or $\frac{1}{4}$-inch) osteotome. Then the graft is removed with curved osteotomes. Breakage of the graft at the physis is prevented by straddling the growth plate with the osteotomes.

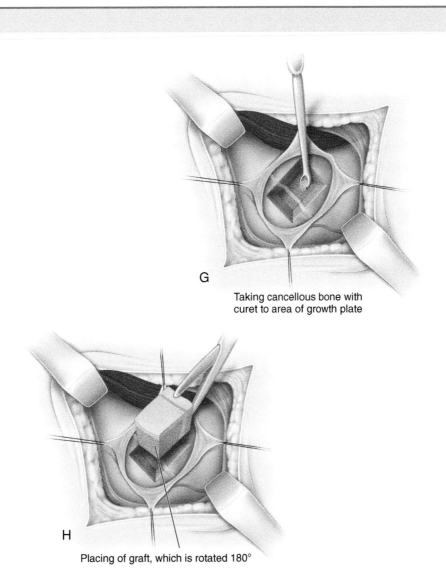

G

Taking cancellous bone with
curet to area of growth plate

H

Placing of graft, which is rotated 180°

G, The growth plate is curetted in anterior, posterior, and distal directions. It should be remembered that the distal femoral physis is pointed inferiorly. The softness of the cartilaginous plate serves as a guide to its direction. Cancellous bone graft is taken from the proximal bed and packed into the defect created by removal of the growth plate.

H, The bone graft is then reinserted into its original bed, with its ends reversed by 180-degree rotation.

Continued on following page

Procedure 52   **Epiphysiodesis of the Distal Femur (the Green Modification of the Phemister Technique), cont'd**

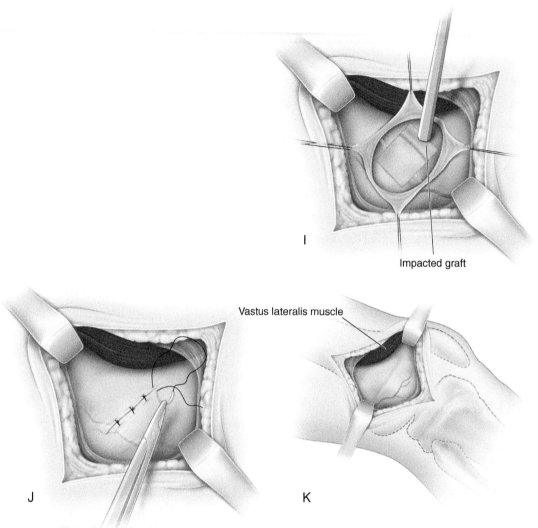

I

Impacted graft

Vastus lateralis muscle

J

Tight closure of periosteum

K

Lateral exposure

I, With an impactor and mallet, the bone graft is securely seated in the bony defect. It should be tapped in a distal direction because the growth plate is inferior in location.

J, The periosteum is tightly closed with interrupted sutures. It is important not to include the patellar retinaculum with the periosteum because doing so will bind it down and thus restrict knee motion. The periosteum is sutured with the knee in complete extension.

K, The same procedure is repeated on the lateral side.

Postoperative Care

A compressive dressing is applied to the wounds. The limb is placed in a knee immobilizer in full extension. In the early postoperative period, the patient should be carefully observed for evidence of excessive swelling leading to a constrictive dressing. This is particularly likely if the patient has undergone a pangeniculate epiphysiodesis or develops acute hemarthrosis. In this event, splitting or loosening of the dressing is necessary.

The patient is started on straight-leg-raising exercises and weight bearing as tolerated with crutches as soon as postsurgical discomfort allows. A patient with significant leg length inequality who does not normally use a shoe lift may need one if walking with the longer leg held straight in the knee immobilizer is too difficult. One week postoperatively, the dressings are removed, and active range-of-motion and strengthening exercises for the knee are instituted. If the patient has a large, uncomfortable hemarthrosis, it should be aspirated; smaller effusions can be ignored. The patient is evaluated between 4 and 6 weeks postoperatively to ensure that full range of motion has been recovered. Patients who are slow to recover knee range of motion may require supervised physical therapy. The patient is allowed to resume normal activities after recovery of knee strength and range of motion, typically 6 to 8 weeks after the surgical procedure.

The patient should be followed radiographically at appropriate intervals until skeletal maturity to document symmetric, complete surgical physeal closure and to monitor the effect of epiphysiodesis on leg length inequality.

Procedure 53   Percutaneous Epiphysiodesis

Operative Technique

The patient is positioned on a radiolucent operating table and the physis is localized by fluoroscopy. **A,** The incision is located over the physis midway between the anterior and posterior surfaces of the femur or tibia. A puncture wound is made with a small blade and a hemostat is used to spread the deeper tissues down to the bone. A drill of ¼ inch diameter is placed against the physis as confirmed by the fluoroscopy. The drill is passed to the center of the tibia or femur and is angulated to remove physeal cartilage anteriorly and posteriorly. Curets, both straight and angled are used to remove the physis with a sweeping motion above and below the physis as seen on the image intensifier. The physis should also be removed anteriorly and posteriorly, taking care not to exit either cortex. **B,** The procedure is done both medially and laterally. If the fibular physis is to be removed, it is done with an anterior incision and direct visualization to avoid peroneal nerve injury **(C).**

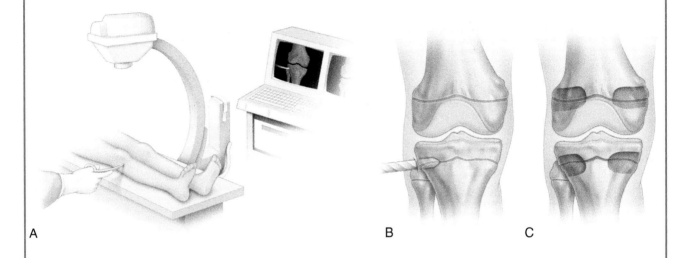

A

B   C

Procedure 54 Epiphysiodesis of the Proximal Tibia and Fibula (the Green Modification of the Phemister Technique)

Operative Technique

A, The patient is placed supine or in a semilateral position. A sterile folded sheet is placed under the knee for support. The knee joint line, the head of the fibula, and the proximal tibial tubercle are identified. A 30-degree slanted oblique incision is made midway between the proximal tibial tubercle and the fibular head; it begins proximally 1 cm inferior to the joint line and 1 cm anterior to the fibular head and extends distally and forward for a distance of 5 cm. The subcutaneous tissue is divided, and the wound flaps are widely undermined and retracted.

B and **C,** The head of the fibula is in line with the proximal growth plate of the tibia. The capsule of the knee joint, the insertion of the biceps tendon, and the fibular collateral ligament of the knee are identified.

The common peroneal nerve lies close to the medial border of the biceps femoris muscle in the popliteal fossa; then it passes distally and laterally between the lateral head of the gastrocnemius and the biceps tendon. Behind the fibular head, the nerve is subcutaneous. At the site of origin of the peroneus longus muscle at the head and neck of the fibula, the common peroneal nerve winds anteriorly around the fibular neck and then passes deep to the peroneus longus muscle and branches into the superficial and deep peroneal nerves.

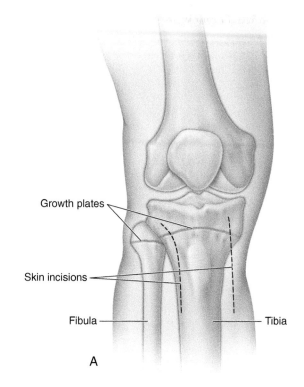

A

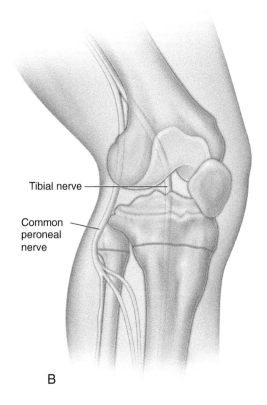

B

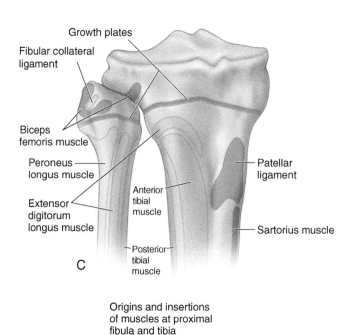

C

Origins and insertions of muscles at proximal fibula and tibia

D, The origins of the toe extensors, extensor hallucis longus, and anterior tibial muscles, along with a cuff of periosteal flap, are elevated from the arcuate line. With a periosteal elevator, the origin of the peroneus longus muscle is detached from the head of the fibula. Keeping the dissection anterior to the fibular head prevents injury to the nerve.

E and F, The site of the growth plate of the proximal fibula is identified. Next a longitudinal incision is made on the anterior aspect of the fibular head and is extended distally to include the growth plate. Alternatively, a rectangular piece of bone (¼ inch wide and ½ inch long) is removed from the proximal fibula, thus straddling the physis. Three fourths of the length of the bone graft includes the fibular head, so that only one fourth of the graft length includes the metaphysis. The growth plate is thoroughly curetted, the ends of the bone graft are reversed (180 degrees), and the piece of bone is placed securely back in the graft bed. I simply curet the growth plate anteriorly to posteriorly.

The lateral aspect of the proximal tibial physis is already exposed for the fibular epiphysiodesis. A longitudinal incision is made midway between the anterior and posterior borders of the lateral tibia. The periosteum is elevated, and a rectangular piece of bone is resected in a manner similar to that described for the bone graft technique in the distal femur. The steps of the epiphysiodesis are the same as those outlined in Procedure 51**G** to **K** for epiphysiodesis of the distal femur.

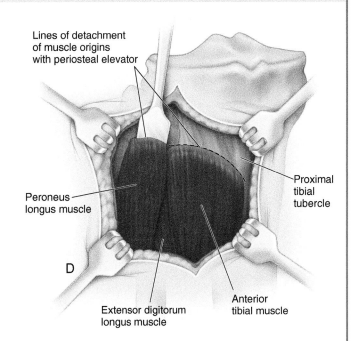

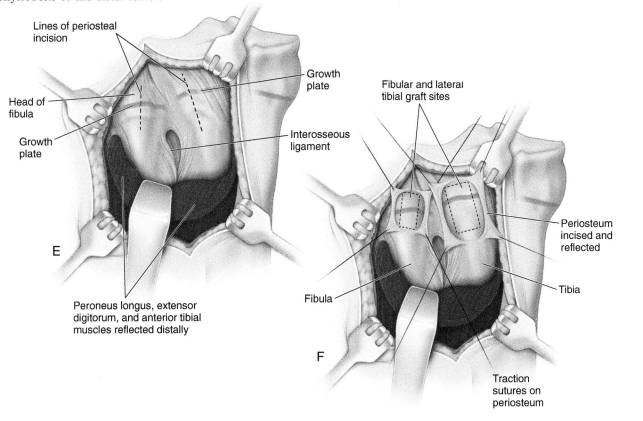

Continued on following page

Procedure 54   Epiphysiodesis of the Proximal Tibia and Fibula (the Green Modification of the Phemister Technique), cont'd

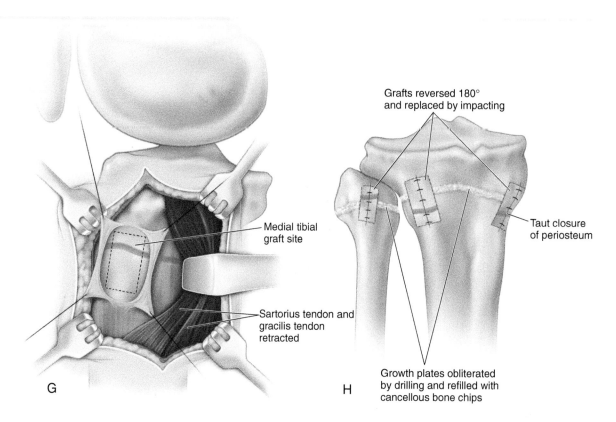

Grafts reversed 180°
and replaced by impacting

Medial tibial
graft site

Taut closure
of periosteum

Sartorius tendon and
gracilis tendon
retracted

Growth plates obliterated
by drilling and refilled with
cancellous bone chips

G

H

G and **H,** The medial side of the proximal tibial physis is exposed by a longitudinal incision approximately 3 cm long, beginning 1 cm distal to the joint line and continuing distally midway between the proximal tibial tubercle and posteromedial margin of the tibia. The subcutaneous tissue and deep fascia are divided in line with the skin incision. The anterior margins of the sartorius tendon and tibial collateral ligament are partially elevated and retracted posteriorly.

The steps for growth arrest of the proximal tibial physis follow the steps described for a distal femoral epiphysiodesis. The rectangular piece of bone graft removed from the tibia, usually ½ inch wide and ¾ inch long, is smaller than that removed from the femur. Before closure of the wound, the tourniquet is released, and hemostasis is secured.

Postoperative Care

After closure of the wound, a compressive dressing and knee immobilizer are applied. Postoperative management is the same as for a distal femoral epiphysiodesis. In general, hemarthrosis is much less likely, and recovery of range of motion is much more rapid and certain after proximal tibial and fibular epiphysiodesis than after distal femoral epiphysiodesis.

Procedure 55   Ischial-Bearing Above-Knee Amputation (Midthigh Amputation)

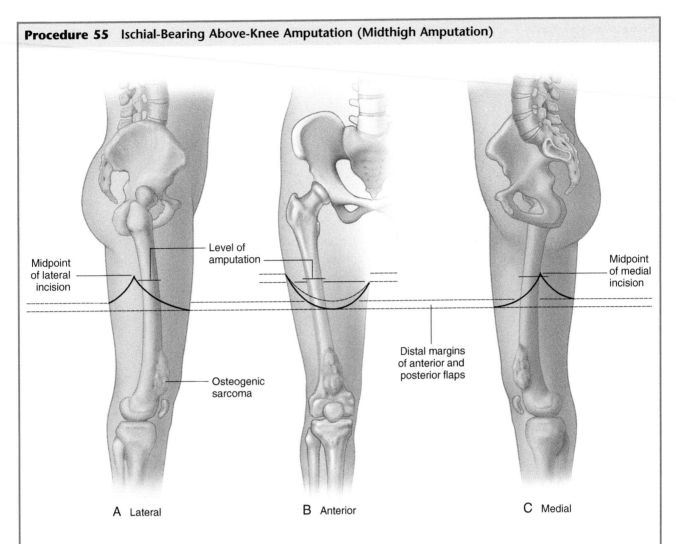

A Lateral   B Anterior   C Medial

The level of amputation is determined by measurements taken from preoperative imaging studies. Measurements are made from the top of the greater trochanter and from the knee joint line. If the level of amputation permits, a pneumatic tourniquet is used for hemostasis. A sandbag is placed under the ipsilateral buttock.

The following areas are marked: 1. Intended bone level of amputation. 2. Midpoints of the medial and lateral aspects of the thigh 1 cm above the bony level. 3. Distal border of the anterior and posterior incisions

The last is determined by a rule of thumb; the combined length of the anterior and posterior flaps is slightly longer than the diameter of the thigh at the intended bone level, and the length of the anterior flap is twice the diameter of the posterior flap.

A to C, The skin incision begins at the midpoint of the medial aspect of the thigh, gently curves anteriorly and inferiorly to the distal border of the anterior incision, and passes convexly to the midpoint on the lateral aspect of the thigh. The posterior incision starts at the same medial point, extends to the distal margin of the posterior flap, and swings proximally to end at the midpoint on the lateral thigh.

Continued on following page

Procedure 55   Ischial-Bearing Above-Knee Amputation (Midthigh Amputation), cont'd

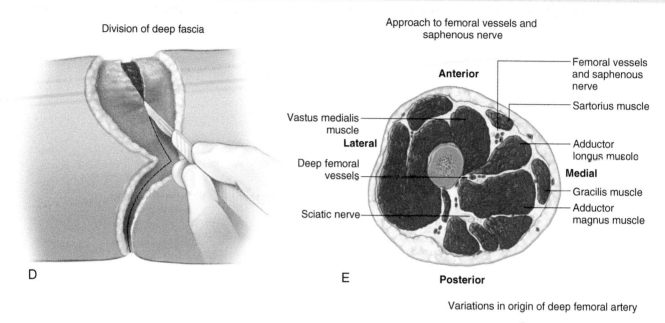

Division of deep fascia

Approach to femoral vessels and saphenous nerve

Anterior

Vastus medialis muscle

Lateral

Deep femoral vessels

Sciatic nerve

Femoral vessels and saphenous nerve

Sartorius muscle

Adductor longus muscle

Medial

Gracilis muscle

Adductor magnus muscle

D

E

Posterior

Variations in origin of deep femoral artery

Line of division of saphenous nerve

Deep fascia retracted

Sartorius muscle retracted laterally

Deep femoral vessels may be ligated and divided through this incision if amputation level is high

Femoral artery and vein doubly ligated and divided

F

Femoral artery

Profunda femoris artery 52%

Femoral artery

Profunda femoris artery 21.8%

Femoral artery

G

Profunda femoris artery 15%

D, The subcutaneous tissue and deep fascia are divided in line with the skin incision, and the anterior and posterior flaps are reflected proximally to the amputation level. **E to G,** The femoral vessels and saphenous nerve are identified. They are located deep to the sartorius muscle, between the adductor longus and vastus medialis muscles. The deep femoral vessels are found adjacent to the femur in the interval between the adductor magnus, adductor longus, and vastus medialis muscles. There are variations in the origin of the deep femoral artery, as shown in **G.** The femoral artery and vein are isolated, doubly ligated with heavy silk sutures, and divided. The saphenous nerve is pulled distally and divided with a sharp scalpel. If the amputation level is high, the deep femoral vessels may be ligated and divided through this anteromedial approach.

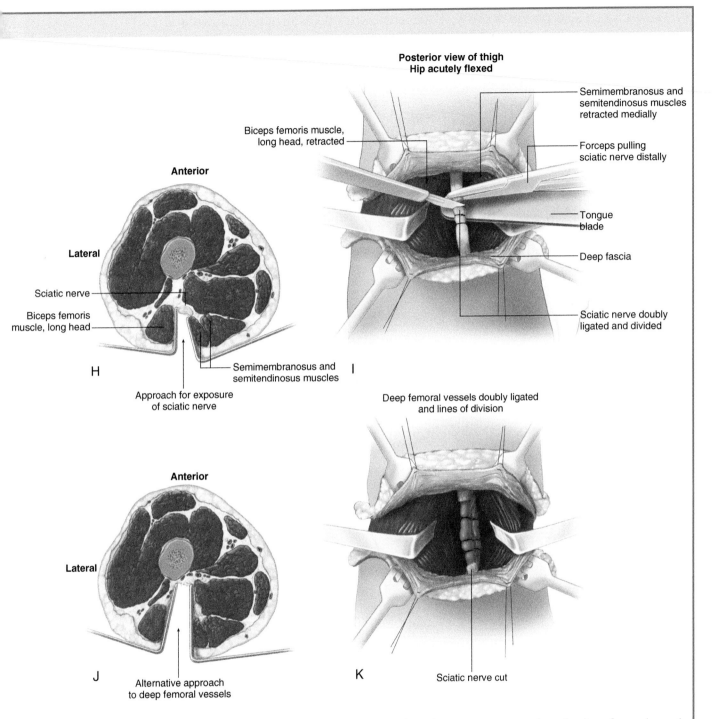

**Posterior view of thigh
Hip acutely flexed**

Biceps femoris muscle, long head, retracted

Semimembranosus and semitendinosus muscles retracted medially

Forceps pulling sciatic nerve distally

Tongue blade

Deep fascia

Sciatic nerve doubly ligated and divided

Anterior

Lateral

Sciatic nerve

Biceps femoris muscle, long head

Semimembranosus and semitendinosus muscles

H

I

Approach for exposure of sciatic nerve

Deep femoral vessels doubly ligated and lines of division

Anterior

Lateral

J

Alternative approach to deep femoral vessels

K

Sciatic nerve cut

H and I, The hip is acutely flexed to approach the posterior structures. The sciatic nerve is exposed in the interval between the medial hamstrings medially and long head of the biceps femoris laterally. The nerve is gently pulled distally, infiltrated with bupivacaine, ligated, and sharply divided over a tongue blade.

J and K, The posterior approach to the deep femoral vessels when the level of amputation is distal is shown.

Continued on following page

Procedure 55   Ischial-Bearing Above-Knee Amputation (Midthigh Amputation), cont'd

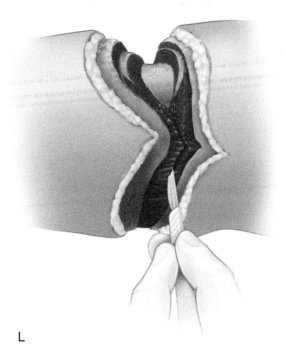

L

Division of muscles

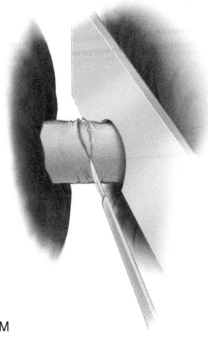

M

Circular incision of periosteum of femur

L, With an amputation knife or electrocautery, the quadriceps and adductor muscles are sectioned and beveled upward to the site of bone division so that the anterior myofascial flap is approximately 1.5 cm thick. The posterior muscles are divided transversely. Muscular branches of the femoral vessels are clamped and ligated as necessary.

M, The proximal muscles are retracted upward with an amputation shield, and the periosteum is incised circumferentially.

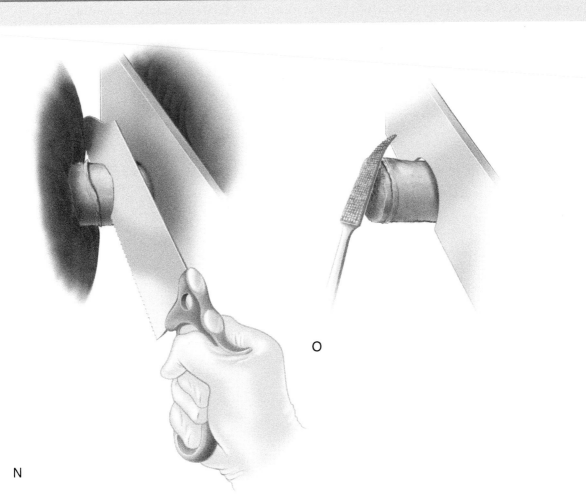

N   O

Femur divided with saw   Irregular bone ends smoothed with rasp

N, The femur is sectioned with a saw immediately distal to the periosteal incision.

O, With a rongeur, the prominence of the linea aspera is excised, and the bone end is smoothed with a file. The wound is irrigated with normal saline solution to wash away all loose fragments of bone.

Continued on following page

Procedure 55   Ischial-Bearing Above-Knee Amputation (Midthigh Amputation), cont'd

Proximal stump

Rectus femoris muscle

Vastus medialis muscle

Vastus intermedius muscle

Vastus lateralis muscle

Biceps femoris muscle, short head

Sciatic nerve

Biceps femoris muscle, long head

Femoral vessels and saphenous nerve

Sartorius muscle

Great saphenous vein

Adductor longus muscle

Deep femoral vessels

Gracilis muscle

Adductor magnus muscle

Semimembranosus muscle

Semitendinosus muscle

P

Closure of deep fascia

Q

Suction catheters

R   Skin edges approximated and closed

P, Hot packs are applied over the wound, and the tourniquet is released. After 5 minutes, the stump is inspected for any bleeders.

Q, The anterior and posterior myofascial flaps are pulled distally and approximated with interrupted sutures through their fascial layer. Suction catheters are placed in the wound and connected to a closed suction drainage evacuator.

R, The subcutaneous tissue and skin are closed in the usual manner. Some centers perform immediate prosthetic fitting in the operating room. Others apply a splint initially and change to compression soft dressings on the second postoperative day.

Procedure 56   Disarticulation of the Knee Joint

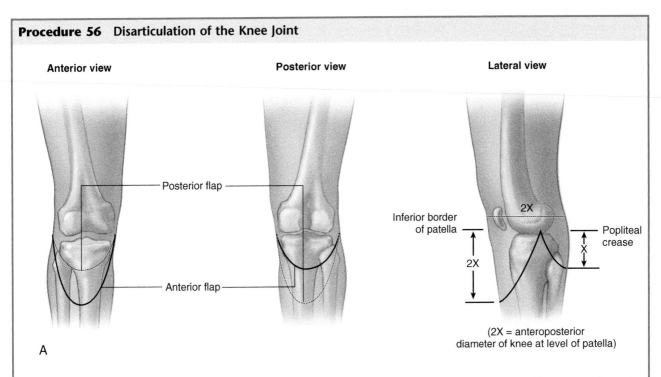

The patient is placed in a lateral position so that he or she can easily be turned to a supine, prone, or semilateral position. The operation is performed using pneumatic tourniquet ischemia.

A, The skin incisions are placed so that a long anterior flap and short posterior flap are provided; thus the operative scar is posterior and away from the weight-bearing skin. Measuring from the distal pole of the patella to the distal border, the length of the anterior flap is equal to the anteroposterior diameter of the knee, whereas the posterior flap is half the length of the anterior flap. The medial and lateral proximal points of the incisions are at the joint line at the junction of the anterior two thirds and posterior third of the diameter of the knee. The anterior and posterior wound flaps are raised, including the subcutaneous tissue and deep fascia.

Continued on following page

Procedure 56   Disarticulation of the Knee Joint, cont'd

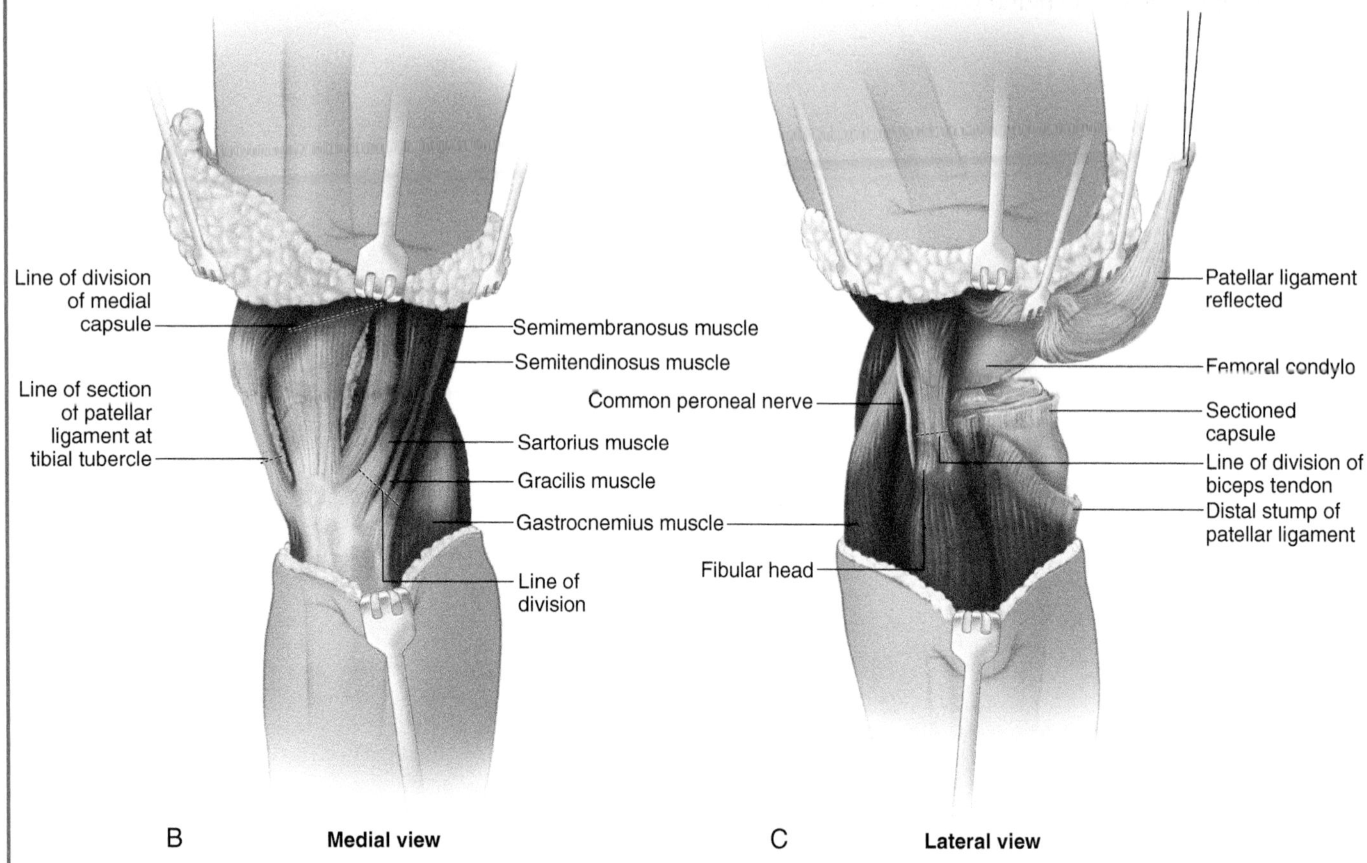

Line of division of medial capsule

Line of section of patellar ligament at tibial tubercle

Semimembranosus muscle

Semitendinosus muscle

Common peroneal nerve

Sartorius muscle

Gracilis muscle

Gastrocnemius muscle

Line of division

B   **Medial view**

Patellar ligament reflected

Femoral condylo

Sectioned capsule

Line of division of biceps tendon

Distal stump of patellar ligament

Fibular head

C   **Lateral view**

B, The medial aspects of the knee joint and the proximal tibia are exposed. Tendons of the sartorius, gracilis, semi-membranosus, and semitendinosus muscles are identified, marked with size 0 silk whip sutures, and sectioned near their insertions on the tibia. The patellar tendon is detached at the proximal tibial tubercle. The anterior and medial joint capsule and synovial membrane are divided proximally near the femoral condyles.

C, The lateral aspect of the knee joint is exposed. The iliotibial tract is divided, and the biceps femoris tendon is sectioned from its attachment to the head of the fibula. The lateral part of the joint capsule and synovial membrane is divided above the joint line.

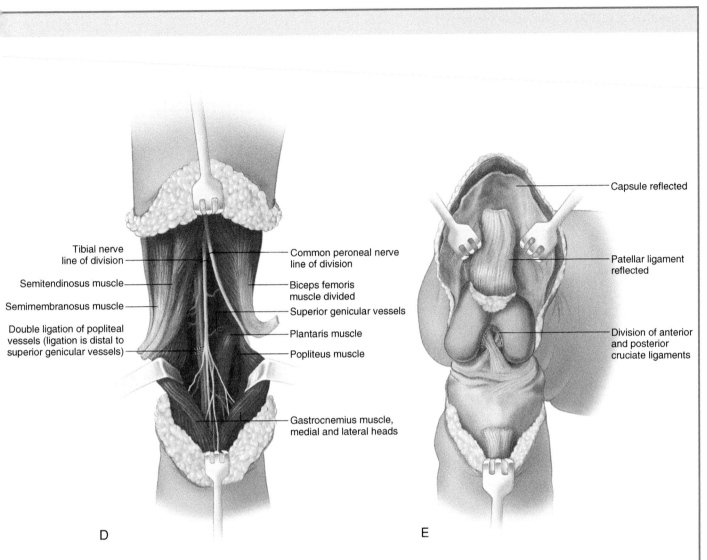

Tibial nerve
line of division

Semitendinosus muscle

Semimembranosus muscle

Double ligation of popliteal
vessels (ligation is distal to
superior genicular vessels)

Common peroneal nerve
line of division

Biceps femoris
muscle divided

Superior genicular vessels

Plantaris muscle

Popliteus muscle

Gastrocnemius muscle,
medial and lateral heads

Capsule reflected

Patellar ligament
reflected

Division of anterior
and posterior
cruciate ligaments

D

E

D, Now the patient is turned to the semiprone position, and the popliteal fossa is exposed. The popliteal vessels are identified by blunt dissection; the popliteal artery and vein are separately doubly ligated distal to the origin of the superior genicular branches and divided. The tibial nerve and common peroneal nerve are pulled distally, sharply divided with a scalpel, and allowed to retract proximally. The medial and lateral heads of the gastrocnemius are extraperiosteally elevated and stripped from the posterior aspect of the femoral condyles. The distal femoral epiphyseal plate should not be damaged. The plantaris and popliteus muscles, oblique popliteal ligament, posterior part of the capsule of the knee joint, and meniscofemoral ligaments are completely divided.

E, The patient is placed in a semisupine position, and the knee is flexed acutely. The cruciate ligaments are identified and sectioned, completing the amputation. The pneumatic tourniquet is released, and complete hemostasis is secured.

Continued on following page

Procedure 56   Disarticulation of the Knee Joint, cont'd

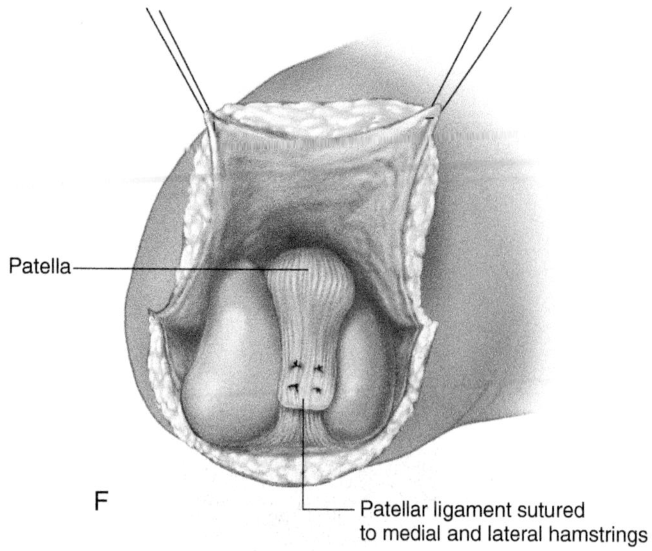

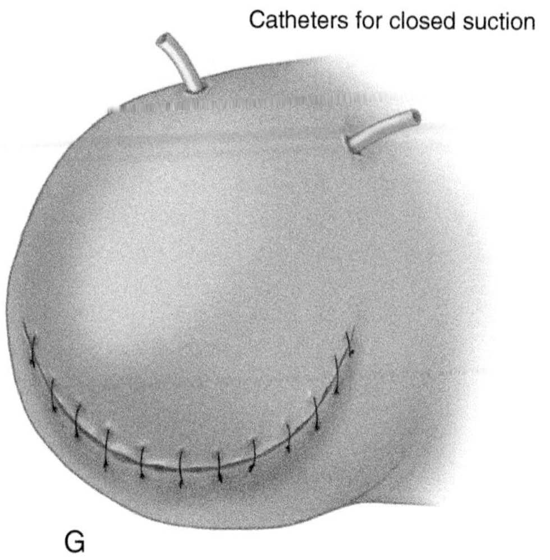

F

Patella

Patellar ligament sutured
to medial and lateral hamstrings

Catheters for closed suction

G

F, The patellar tendon is sutured to the medial and lateral hamstrings in the intercondylar notch. In children, the patella usually is not removed, and reshaping of the femoral condyles should not be performed because of the danger of damaging the growth plate. Synovectomy is not indicated.

G, Two catheters are placed in the wound for closed suction. The deep fascia and subcutaneous tissue of the anterior and posterior flaps are approximated with interrupted sutures, and the skin is closed in routine fashion.

Procedure 57   Below-Knee Amputation

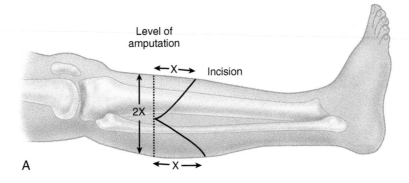

Level of amputation

←X→   Incision

2X

A

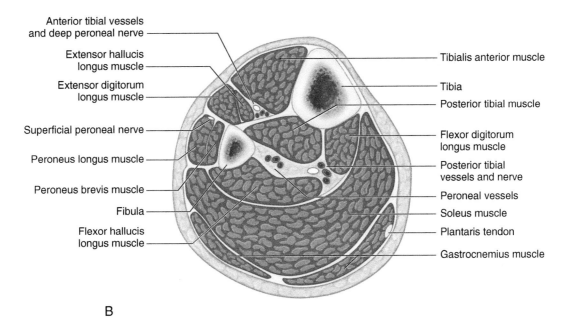

Anterior tibial vessels
and deep peroneal nerve

Extensor hallucis
longus muscle

Extensor digitorum
longus muscle

Superficial peroneal nerve

Peroneus longus muscle

Peroneus brevis muscle

Fibula

Flexor hallucis
longus muscle

Tibialis anterior muscle

Tibia

Posterior tibial muscle

Flexor digitorum
longus muscle

Posterior tibial
vessels and nerve

Peroneal vessels

Soleus muscle

Plantaris tendon

Gastrocnemius muscle

B

The level of amputation is determined preoperatively. With the patient supine, a pneumatic tourniquet is applied on the proximal thigh.

A and **B,** The line of incision for the anterior and posterior flaps is marked on the skin, and the anteroposterior diameter of the leg at the level of bone section is measured.

The anterior flap can be fashioned slightly longer than the posterior flap, or they may be of equal length, because the position of the scar is not important in terms of prosthetic fitting. The length of each flap is half the anteroposterior diameter of the leg.

Continued on following page

Procedure 57   Below-Knee Amputation, cont'd

Level of sectioning
superficial
peroneal nerve

Extensor digitorum
longus muscle

Peroneus
brevis muscle

Anterior tibial
vessels

Deep peroneal nerve

Extensor hallucis
longus muscle

C   **Anterior view**

D   **Posterior view**

Oblique cut of anteromedial
tibial cortex

Peroneus
muscles

Triceps surae muscle Fibula

Transverse cut of tibia

Fibula

E

F

C and D, The incisions are deepened to the deep fascia, which is divided in line with the skin incision. The anterior and posterior flaps are raised proximally in one layer, including skin, subcutaneous tissue, and deep fascia. Over the anteromedial surface of the tibia, the periosteum is incised with the deep fascia, and both are elevated as a continuous layer to the intended level of amputation.

In the interval between the extensor digitorum longus and peroneus brevis muscles, the superficial peroneal nerve is identified; the nerve is pulled distally, sharply divided, and allowed to retract proximally well above the end of the stump.

The anterior tibial vessels and deep peroneal nerve are identified, doubly ligated, and divided.

E and F, The muscles in the anterior tibial compartment are sectioned approximately 0.75 cm distal to the level of bone section. The tibial crest is beveled as follows: Beginning 2 cm proximal to the level of amputation, a 45-degree distal oblique cut is made, ending 0.5 cm anterior to the medullary cavity.

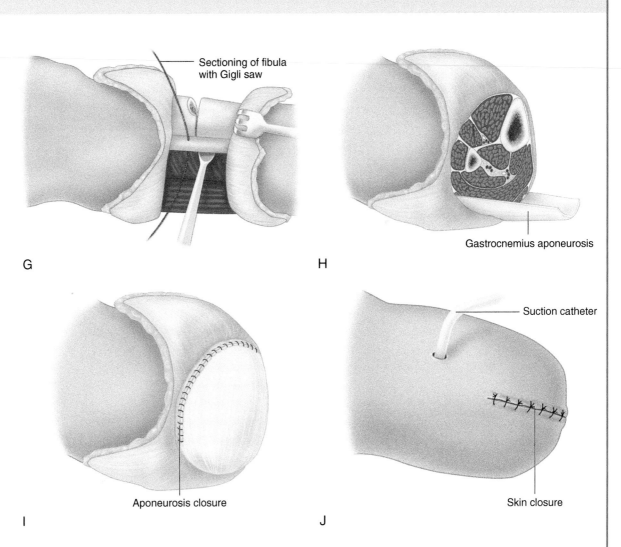

G, The tibia is transversely sectioned. The angle of division should be at a right angle to the axis of the bone.

H, The fibula is cleared of surrounding muscle and, using a Gigli saw, sectioned 2 to 3 cm proximal to the distal end of the tibia. The bone ends are smoothed and rounded with a rasp. All periosteal fringes are excised, and the wound is irrigated with normal saline solution to remove bone dust.

Next, the posterior muscles in the leg are sectioned. The posterior tibial and peroneal vessels are carefully identified, doubly ligated, and divided. The tibial nerve is pulled distally and divided with a sharp knife. A fascial flap is developed from the gastrocnemius aponeurosis so that it can be brought forward to cover the end of the stump.

I and J, The tourniquet is released following application of hot laparotomy pads and pressure over the cut surfaces of the muscles and bones. After 5 minutes, the pads are removed, and complete hemostasis is secured. The wound should be completely dry. The fascia of the gastrocnemius muscle is brought anteriorly and sutured to the fascia of the anterior compartment muscles. The muscles may be partially excised if they are bulky at the side of the stump. Suction drainage catheters are placed deep to the gastrocnemius fascia. The subcutaneous tissue and skin are closed with interrupted sutures. A nonadherent dressing and splint are applied; alternatively, an immediate fit prosthesis can be applied.

Procedure 58   **Arthrodesis of the Ankle Joint via the Anterior Approach Without Disturbing the Distal Tibial Growth Plate**

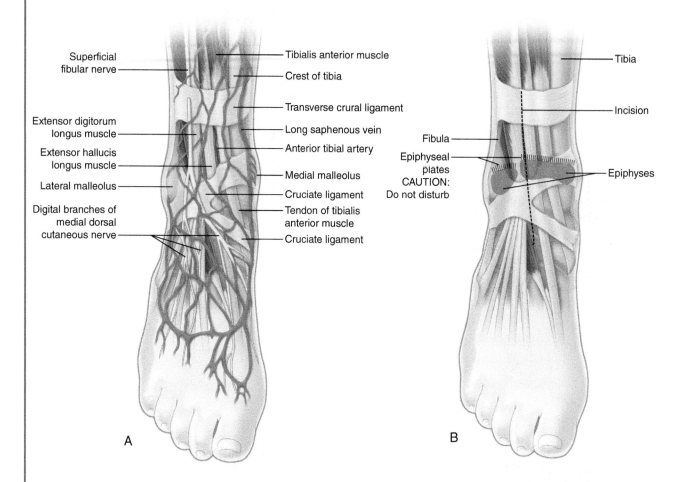

A

B

Operative Technique

A and **B,** A longitudinal skin incision is made beginning 7 cm proximal to the ankle joint between the extensor digitorum longus and extensor hallucis longus tendons and extended distally across the ankle joint in line with the third metatarsal; the incision ends 4 cm distal to the ankle joint.

The subcutaneous tissue is divided and the skin flaps are mobilized and retracted to their respective sides. The veins crossing the field are clamped, divided, and coagulated. The intermediate and medial dorsal cutaneous branches of the superficial peroneal nerve are identified and protected by retraction to one side of the wound.

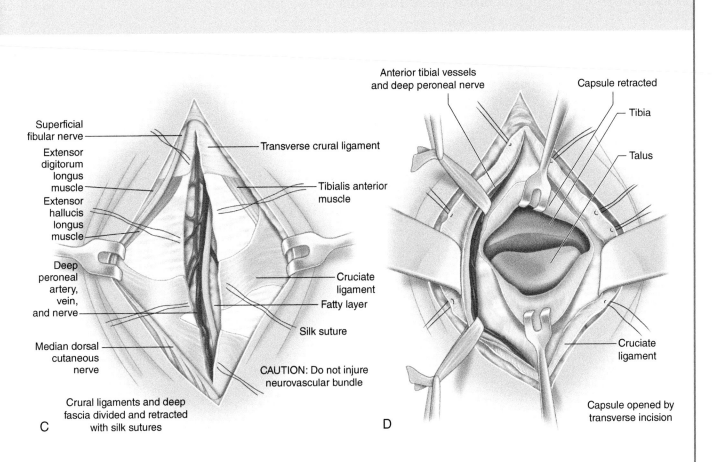

Superficial
fibular nerve

Extensor
digitorum
longus
muscle

Extensor
hallucis
longus
muscle

Deep
peroneal
artery,
vein,
and nerve

Median dorsal
cutaneous
nerve

Transverse crural ligament

Tibialis anterior
muscle

Cruciate
ligament

Fatty layer

Silk suture

CAUTION: Do not injure
neurovascular bundle

Crural ligaments and deep
fascia divided and retracted
with silk sutures

C

Anterior tibial vessels
and deep peroneal nerve

Capsule retracted

Tibia

Talus

Cruciate
ligament

Capsule opened by
transverse incision

D

C, The deep fascia and transverse crural and cruciate crural ligaments are divided in line with the skin incision. The ligaments are marked with 00 silk suture for accurate closure later.

D, The neurovascular bundle (deep peroneal nerve, anterior tibial–dorsalis pedis vessels) is identified, isolated, and retracted laterally with the extensor hallucis longus, extensor digitorum longus, and peroneus tertius tendons. The anterolateral malleolar and lateral tarsal arteries are isolated, clamped, divided, and ligated. The distal end of the tibia, ankle joint, and talus are identified. A transverse incision is made in the capsule of the talotibial joint from the posterior tip of the medial malleolus to the lateral malleolus. The edges of the capsule are marked with 00 silk suture for meticulous closure later.

Continued on following page

Procedure 58   Arthrodesis of the Ankle Joint via the Anterior Approach Without Disturbing
the Distal Tibial Growth Plate, cont'd

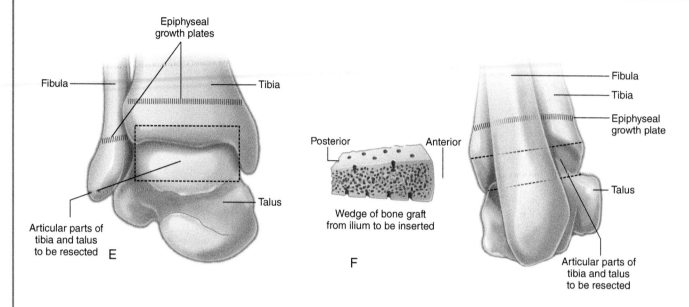

Epiphyseal
growth plates

Fibula

Tibia

Articular parts of
tibia and talus
to be resected   E

Talus

Posterior   Anterior

Wedge of bone graft
from ilium to be inserted

F

Fibula

Tibia

Epiphyseal
growth plate

Talus

Articular parts of
tibia and talus
to be resected

E to G, The capsule is reflected and retracted distally
on the talus and proximally on the tibia. The periosteum
of the tibia should not be divided. The distal tibial and
fibular epiphyseal plates should not be disturbed in
growing children. With thin curved and straight osteotomes, the cartilage and subchondral bone are removed
from the opposing articular surfaces of the distal tibia
and proximal talus down to raw bleeding cancellous
bone. Cartilage chips should not be left posteriorly.

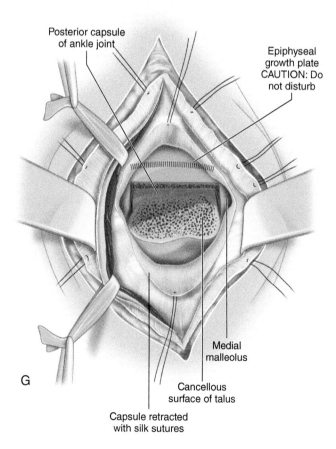

Posterior capsule
of ankle joint

Epiphyseal
growth plate
CAUTION: Do
not disturb

Medial
malleolus

G

Cancellous
surface of talus

Capsule retracted
with silk sutures

H, Next a large piece of bone for grafting is taken from the ilium and fashioned to fit snugly in the ankle joint. The graft should have both cortices intact and should be thicker at one end and wedge shaped. The cortices of the graft are perforated with multiple tiny drill holes. The ankle joint is held in the desired position, and the bone graft is firmly fitted into the joint with an impactor. If any space is left on each side of the graft, it is packed with cancellous bone from the ilium. The graft in the ankle joint gives compression force to the arthrodesis and adds to the height of the foot and ankle. The capsule of the ankle joint and the transverse crural and cruciate crural ligaments are closed carefully in layers. The deep fascia and the wound are closed in the usual manner. Anteroposterior and lateral radiographs are taken to ensure that the ankle joint is in the desired position.

I, A long-leg cast is applied with the ankle joint in the desired position of plantar flexion (boys, 10 degrees; girls, 15 to 20 degrees) and the knee in 45 degrees of flexion.

Postoperative Care

Periodic radiographs are taken to determine the position of the graft and the extent of healing. Eight to 10 weeks after surgery, the solid cast is removed and radiographs are taken with the cast off. Ordinarily, by this time the fusion is solid and the patient is gradually allowed to be ambulatory. Full weight bearing is begun 2 to 3 weeks later.

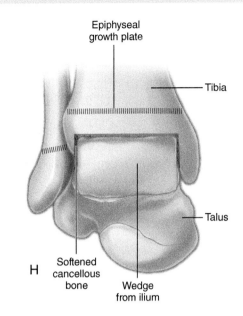

Epiphyseal growth plate

Tibia

Talus

H Softened cancellous bone

Wedge from ilium

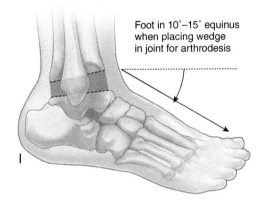

Foot in 10°–15° equinus when placing wedge in joint for arthrodesis

I

SECTION V

UPPER EXTREMITY DISORDERS

Several procedures are useful to improve function for the child with a brachial plexus palsy. In late cases, lateral rotational osteotomy can place the upper extremity in a more functional position. Likewise, in late cases, the Zancolli procedure changes the function of the biceps from being a supinator to that of a pronator of the forearm. This is useful when there is a recalcitrant supination contracture.

Sprengel's deformity consists of congenitally elevated scapula that is tethered to the thorax with a loss of scapula-thoracic mobility. Surgery reduces the deformity by lowering the scapula and removing a portion of the upper scapular bone. Freeing the fibrous tethers to the spine and thorax allows the scapula to move more freely, but some restriction will usually persist.

Procedure 59   Lateral Rotation Osteotomy of the Humerus

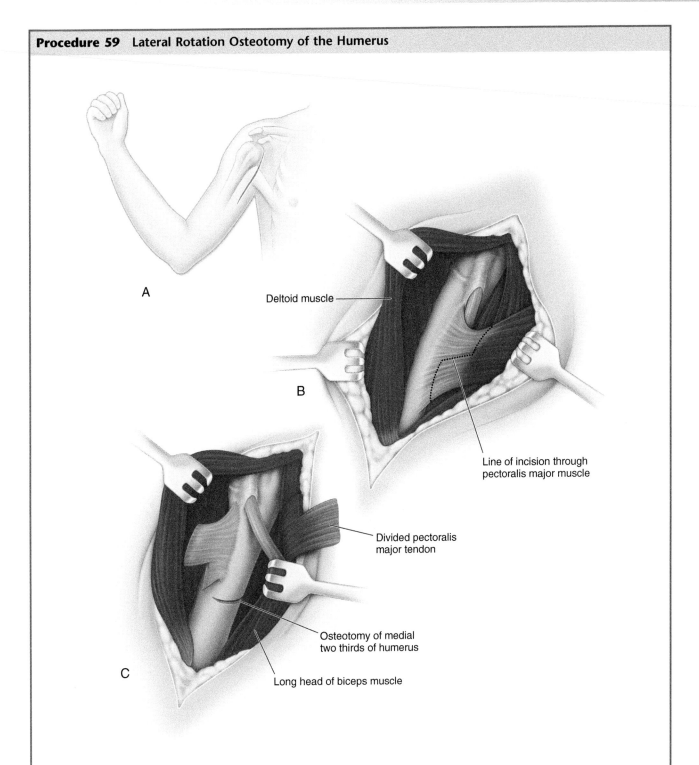

Deltoid muscle

Line of incision through
pectoralis major muscle

B

Divided pectoralis
major tendon

Osteotomy of medial
two thirds of humerus

Long head of biceps muscle

C

Operative Technique

A, The skin incision begins at the coracoid process, extends to the middle of the axilla, curves distally on the medial aspect of the arm, and terminates at its upper third. Surgical exposure of the proximal end of the humerus by this axillary approach results in minimal visibility of the operative scar.

B, The lateral skin margin is retracted laterally. With the shoulder in medial rotation, the upper humeral shaft is exposed. The surgeon must avoid injury to the cephalic vein and anterior humeral circumflex vessels. The proximal humeral physis should not be disturbed.

C, The level of osteotomy is distal to the insertion of the pectoralis major and proximal to the insertion of the deltoid.

Continued on following page

Procedure 59   Lateral Rotation Osteotomy of the Humerus, cont'd

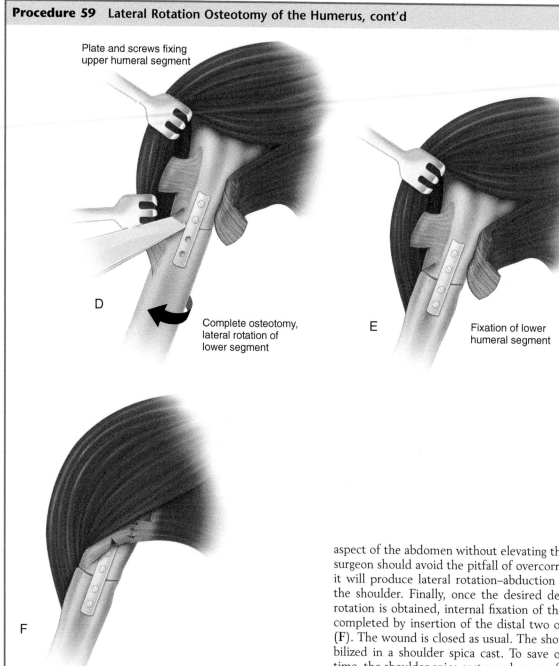

Plate and screws fixing
upper humeral segment

D

Complete osteotomy,
lateral rotation of
lower segment

E

Fixation of lower
humeral segment

F

D to F, This increases range of shoulder abduction and also facilitates exposure of the humeral shaft. We recommend internal fixation with a four- or five-hole plate. First, the surgeon performs an incomplete osteotomy of the humeral diaphysis three fourths of the way through the anteromedial aspect. Second, the humeral segment is fixed to the plate with two screws (**D**). The osteotomy is completed with an electric saw, and the arm is rotated laterally to the desired degree and temporarily fixed with bone-holding forceps (**E**). Next, passive range of shoulder rotation is tested. The ideal position of the shoulder is complete lateral rotation in 90 degrees of abduction. Then, with the shoulder in adduction, the hand should touch the anterior aspect of the abdomen without elevating the scapula. The surgeon should avoid the pitfall of overcorrection because it will produce lateral rotation–abduction contracture of the shoulder. Finally, once the desired degree of lateral rotation is obtained, internal fixation of the osteotomy is completed by insertion of the distal two or three screws (**F**). The wound is closed as usual. The shoulder is immobilized in a shoulder spica cast. To save operating room time, the shoulder spica cast may be manufactured before surgery, bivalved, and fitted at the completion of surgery.

Postoperative Care

Six weeks after surgery the cast is removed and range-of-motion exercises of the shoulder and elbow are performed.

The results of lateral rotation osteotomy of the humerus are very satisfactory; the improved rotational posture of the shoulder increases range of shoulder abduction.

Anterior dislocation of the radial head may be minimized by transfer of the biceps tendon to the brachialis tendon and an attempt at reduction. Posterior dislocation of the radial head is best addressed at the time that symptoms develop and can be treated by resection.

Procedure 60   **Rerouting of the Biceps Brachii Tendon to Convert Its Motion From Supinator to Pronator of the Forearm (Zancolli Procedure)**

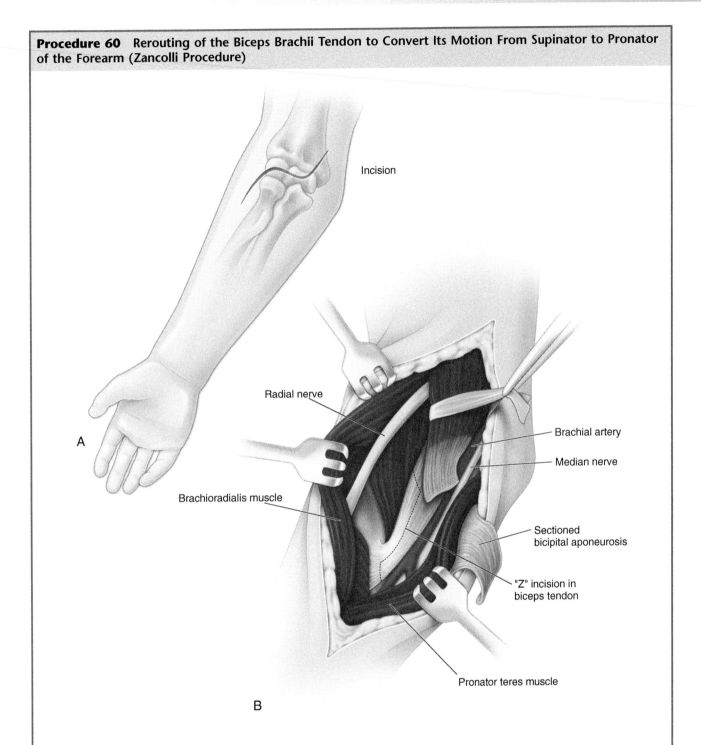

Operative Technique

A, An S-shaped incision is made on the volar surface of the elbow. The incision is begun 3 to 5 cm above the elbow joint and extended to the antecubital crease and then laterally to the radial head and distally into the forearm for a distance of 5 cm. The subcutaneous tissue and deep fascia are divided in line with the skin incision.
B, The biceps tendon is exposed and traced distally to its insertion into the bicipital tuberosity of the radius. The brachial vessels and median nerve are identified and traced.

C, A long Z-plasty of the biceps tendon is performed.
D, The distal segment of the biceps tendon is rerouted around the neck of the radius and passes it mediolaterally.
E, The divided biceps tendon segments are resutured side to side at a length that will maintain full pronation of the forearm and extension of the elbow.

The surgeon should avoid excessive tension on the tendon in young children and when the forearm is hyper-flexible into pronation. The wounds are closed in routine fashion. An above-elbow cast is applied with the elbow in 30 degrees of flexion and the forearm in full pronation.

Continued on following page

Procedure 60   Rerouting of the Biceps Brachii Tendon to Convert Its Motion From Supinator to Pronator of the Forearm (Zancolli Procedure), cont'd

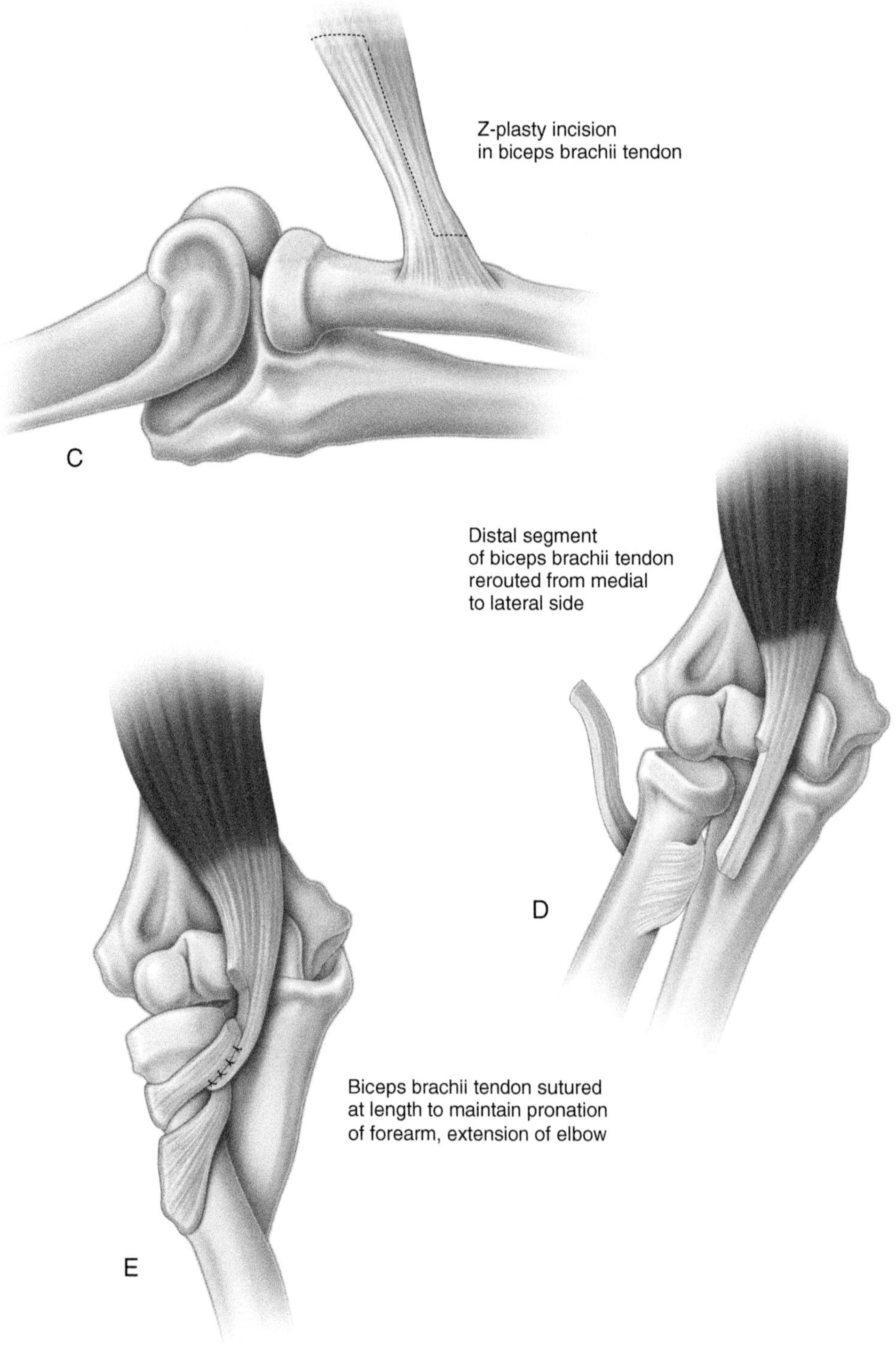

Z-plasty incision
in biceps brachii tendon

C

Distal segment
of biceps brachii tendon
rerouted from medial
to lateral side

D

Biceps brachii tendon sutured
at length to maintain pronation
of forearm, extension of elbow

E

Postoperative Care

Four weeks after surgery the cast is removed, and active assisted exercises are performed three to four times per day to develop pronation and supination of the forearm and elbow flexion–extension. Gentle passive exercises are carried out to maintain full pronation and supination of the forearm and complete flexion and extension of the elbow. At night a plastic splint is worn to maintain the forearm in full pronation and the elbow in 30 degrees of flexion.

Procedure 61   Modified Green Scapuloplasty for Congenital High Scapula (Sprengel Deformity)

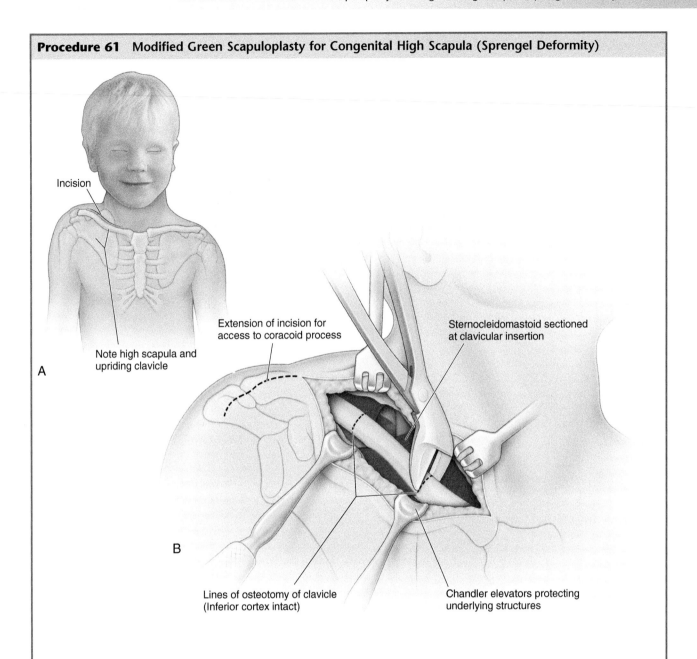

Incision

Note high scapula and
upriding clavicle

A

Extension of incision for
access to coracoid process

Sternocleidomastoid sectioned
at clavicular insertion

B

Lines of osteotomy of clavicle
(Inferior cortex intact)

Chandler elevators protecting
underlying structures

First, an osteotomy of the clavicle is performed. The patient is placed in the lateral decubitus position, and the upper half of the chest, the entire neck, the entire upper limb, and the posterior aspect of the neck are fully prepared and draped. It is vital that the level of the contralateral normal scapula be visible during surgery. An alternative method is to place the patient in the supine position and prepare the neck and upper half of the chest, perform the osteotomy of the clavicle, and then turn the patient to the prone position and reprepare and redrape. This author finds it expedient to use the former method.

Operative Technique

A, A supraclavicular curvilinear incision is made 2 cm above the clavicle in line with the skin creases of the neck and centered over the midportion of the clavicle. It is best to make the skin incision with the neck in slight flexion (not hyperextension). The subcutaneous tissue is divided in line with the skin incision, and the wound is pulled down directly over the clavicle.

B, The deep fascia is incised; any superficial veins are clamped and coagulated. The periosteum of the clavicle is divided longitudinally on its anterior aspect and, with a periosteal elevator, is gently elevated circumferentially around the clavicle. Two smaller Chandler elevators are placed deep to the clavicle to protect the subclavicular vessels and the brachial plexus.

Continued on following page

Procedure 61 Modified Green Scapuloplasty for Congenital High Scapula (Sprengel Deformity), cont'd

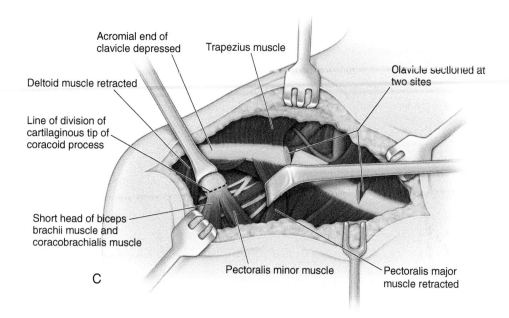

Acromial end of
clavicle depressed

Trapezius muscle

Clavicle sectioned at
two sites

Deltoid muscle retracted

Line of division of
cartilaginous tip of
coracoid process

Short head of biceps
brachii muscle and
coracobrachialis muscle

Pectoralis minor muscle

Pectoralis major
muscle retracted

C

C, With a bone cutter or an oscillating electric saw, the clavicle is sectioned at one or two sites with its posteroinferior cortex left intact (if two sites are used, they should be 3 cm apart). Then by gentle force, a greenstick fracture of the clavicle is produced. The periosteum is closed. The skin is closed with subcuticular running suture. Morcellation of the clavicle is not recommended.

In an older patient the incision may be extended laterally so that the tip of the coracoid process and the origins of the short head of the biceps brachii and the coracobrachialis muscles are exposed. The cartilaginous tip of the coracoid process is sectioned, and then the wound is closed as already described. The purpose of this step in a child older than 10 years is to prevent compression of the neurovascular bundle against the rib.

D, The patient is turned to the prone position with the head and neck extending beyond the operating table and supported on a headrest. The chin piece of the headrest should be well padded, and during the procedure the anesthesiologist should frequently check the chin for pressure areas. Anchoring the buttocks to the operating table with 2- or 3-inch-wide adhesive tape will prevent the patient from slipping caudally. Care should be taken to guard the sterility of the operating field. First, the vertebral border, the level of the inferior angle and the spine of the elevated scapula, and those of the opposite normal scapula are palpated and marked with indelible ink. A midline skin incision is made that begins at the spinous process of the fourth cervical vertebra and extends distally to terminate at the spinous process of the tenth dorsal vertebra (C4 to T10).

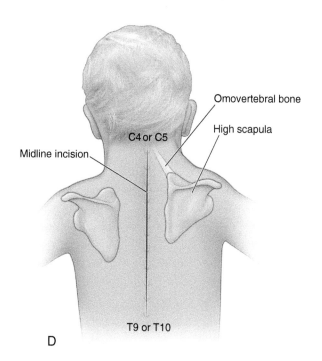

Omovertebral bone

High scapula

C4 or C5

Midline incision

T9 or T10

D

E, The skin and subcutaneous tissue are divided in line with the skin incision, and a place between the subcutaneous tissue and fascia underlying the trapezius muscle is developed. Dissection is extended laterally to expose the spine of the scapula. Next, the inferior margin of the trapezius muscle, which runs obliquely upward and laterally to the scapular spine, is isolated. Its free lateral border is mobilized and retracted proximally and medially. The insertion of the entire trapezius muscle (superior, middle, and inferior parts) on the scapular spine is sectioned, elevated extraperiosteally, and marked with 2-0 Mersilene suture. Inferiorly, the lower fibers of the trapezius muscle are separated from the subjacent latissimus dorsi muscle with Metzenbaum scissors.

F, The detached trapezius muscle is reflected medially to expose the underlying muscles and scapula. The spinal accessory nerve, which is the motor nerve of the trapezius, should not be injured.

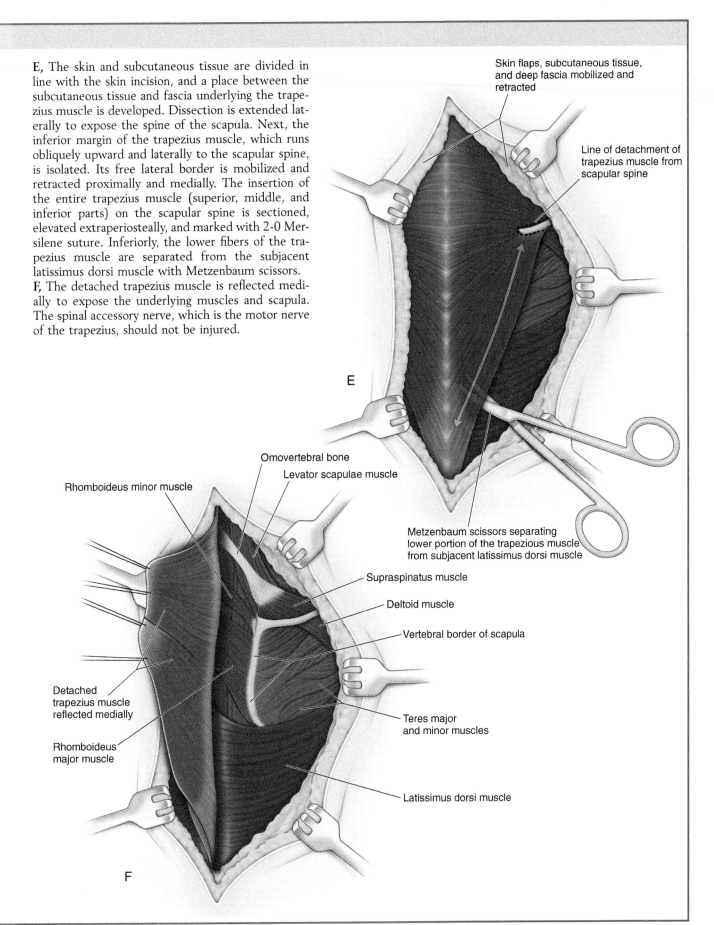

Skin flaps, subcutaneous tissue, and deep fascia mobilized and retracted

Line of detachment of trapezius muscle from scapular spine

Metzenbaum scissors separating lower portion of the trapezious muscle from subjacent latissimus dorsi muscle

E

Omovertebral bone

Levator scapulae muscle

Rhomboideus minor muscle

Supraspinatus muscle

Deltoid muscle

Vertebral border of scapula

Detached trapezius muscle reflected medially

Teres major and minor muscles

Rhomboideus major muscle

Latissimus dorsi muscle

F

Continued on following page

Procedure 61   Modified Green Scapuloplasty for Congenital High Scapula (Sprengel Deformity), cont'd

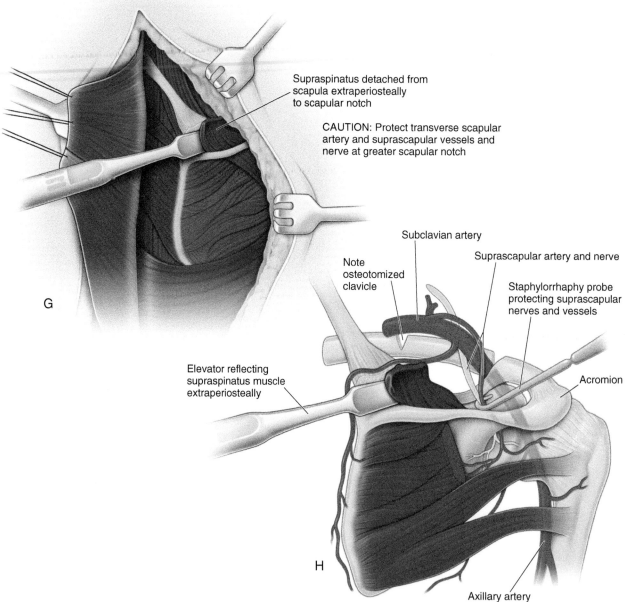

Supraspinatus detached from
scapula extraperiosteally
to scapular notch

CAUTION: Protect transverse scapular
artery and suprascapular vessels and
nerve at greater scapular notch

Subclavian artery

Note
osteotomized
clavicle

Suprascapular artery and nerve

Staphylorrhaphy probe
protecting suprascapular
nerves and vessels

Elevator reflecting
supraspinatus muscle
extraperiosteally

Acromion

G

H

Axillary artery

G and **H,** The supraspinatus muscle is then detached from the scapula extraperiosteally to the greater scapular notch. The transverse scapular artery and suprascapular vessels and nerve must be identified and protected in the lateral portion of the wound as they enter the infraspinatus fossa and pass through the greater scapular notch.

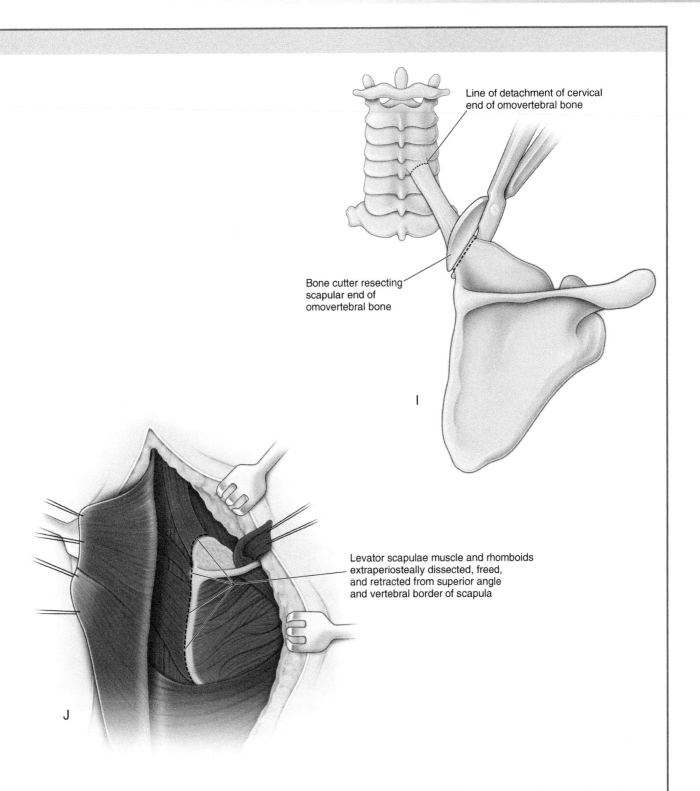

Line of detachment of cervical end of omovertebral bone

Bone cutter resecting scapular end of omovertebral bone

I

Levator scapulae muscle and rhomboids extraperiosteally dissected, freed, and retracted from superior angle and vertebral border of scapula

J

I, The omovertebral bar (bony, cartilaginous, or fibrous) is excised by first sectioning it at the scapular end with a bone cutter and then gently detaching its attachment to the cervical vertebra. At the cervical level it may be attached to the spinous process, lamina, or transverse process of one of the lower cervical vertebrae (fourth to seventh).

J, The insertion of the levator scapulae muscle on the superior angle of the scapula and the insertions of the rhomboideus muscles, major and minor, on the medial border of the scapula are extraperiosteally dissected, divided, and retracted, and their free ends are marked with 2-0 Mersilene suture.

Continued on following page

Procedure 61   Modified Green Scapuloplasty for Congenital High Scapula (Sprengel Deformity), cont'd

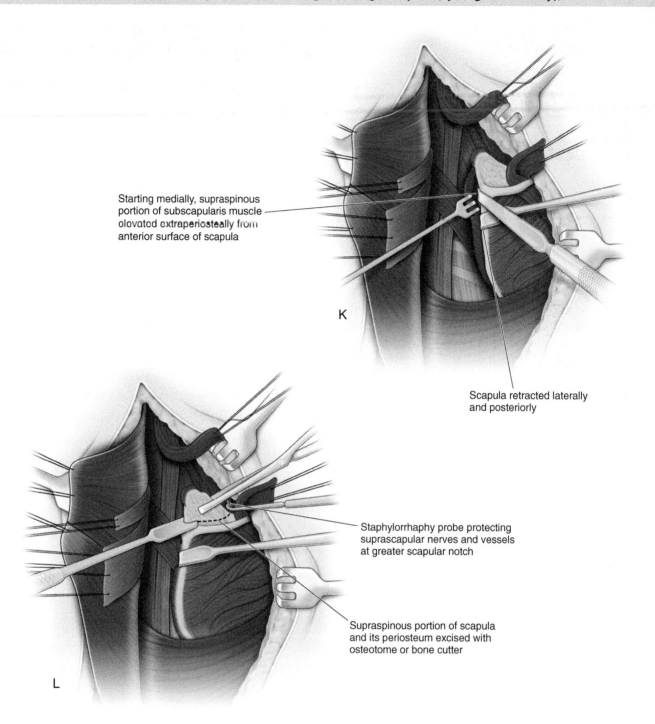

Starting medially, supraspinous portion of subscapularis muscle elevated extraperiosteally from anterior surface of scapula

K

Scapula retracted laterally and posteriorly

Staphylorrhaphy probe protecting suprascapular nerves and vessels at greater scapular notch

Supraspinous portion of scapula and its periosteum excised with osteotome or bone cutter

L

K, The superior margin of the scapula is then retracted posteriorly, and starting medially, the supraspinous portion of the subscapularis muscle is elevated extraperiosteally from the anterior surface of the scapula.

L, Next, a staphylorrhaphy probe is placed in the scapular notch to protect the suprascapular nerves and vessels, and with bone-cutting forceps or an osteotome, the supraspinous part of the scapula along with its periosteum is excised. (Currently, this author preserves the normal anatomy of the scapula because its supraspinous portion is often tilted anteriorly toward the rib cage, in which case a greenstick fracture is produced and the tilted portion elevated.)

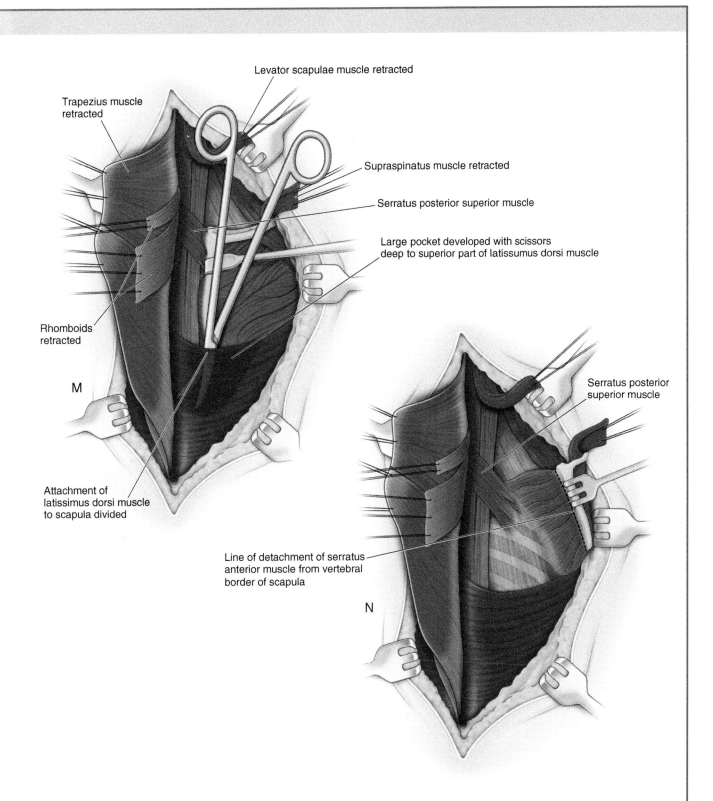

M, The attachments of the latissimus dorsi muscle to the scapula are then divided extraperiosteally, and by blunt dissection a large pocket is created deep to the superior part of the latissimus dorsi muscle.

N, The medial border of the scapula is everted by retracting it posteriorly and laterally, and the insertions of the serratus anterior muscle to the vertebral margin and to the angle of the scapula are freed extraperiosteally and marked with 2-0 Mersilene suture.

Continued on following page

Procedure 61   **Modified Green Scapuloplasty for Congenital High Scapula (Sprengel Deformity), cont'd**

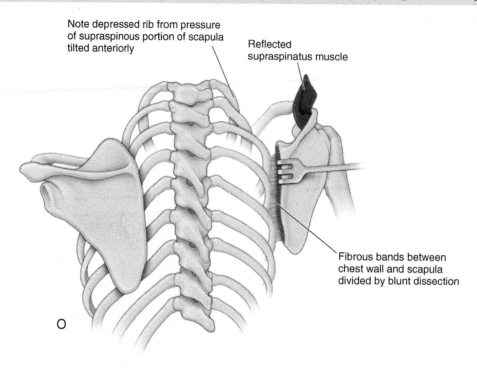

Note depressed rib from pressure
of supraspinous portion of scapula
tilted anteriorly

Reflected
supraspinatus muscle

Fibrous bands between
chest wall and scapula
divided by blunt dissection

O

O, Thick fibrous bands may connect the scapula to the chest
wall. They should be divided to mobilize the scapula so that
it can be displaced distally enough.

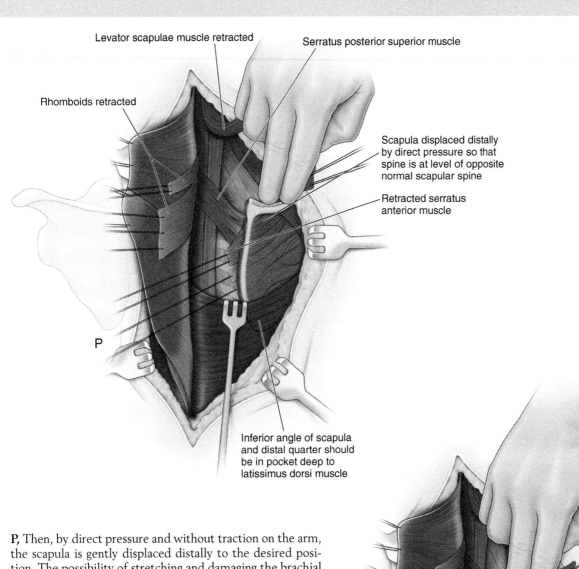

Levator scapulae muscle retracted

Serratus posterior superior muscle

Rhomboids retracted

Scapula displaced distally
by direct pressure so that
spine is at level of opposite
normal scapular spine

Retracted serratus
anterior muscle

P

Inferior angle of scapula
and distal quarter should
be in pocket deep to
latissimus dorsi muscle

P, Then, by direct pressure and without traction on the arm, the scapula is gently displaced distally to the desired position. The possibility of stretching and damaging the brachial plexus must always be kept in mind, and vigorous manipulations should be avoided. The inferior angle and distal quarter of the scapula should be in the large pocket deep to the superior part of the latissimus dorsi muscle.

Q, If winging of the scapula is present, the inferior pole of the scapula is attached to the adjacent rib with two or three absorbable sutures. If the rhomboid muscles and other scapulocostal muscles are hypoplastic or fibrotic and marked winging of the scapula is noted, this author recommends fixing the scapula on the rib cage in a lowered and more laterally rotated position. The winging will be corrected, and the laterally rotated fixed position of the scapula will enable the patient to abduct the shoulder fully at the glenohumeral joint.

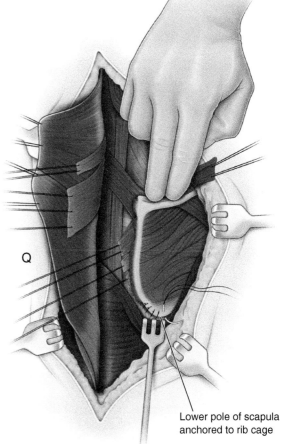

Q

Lower pole of scapula
anchored to rib cage

Continued on following page

Procedure 61   Modified Green Scapuloplasty for Congenital High Scapula (Sprengel Deformity), cont'd

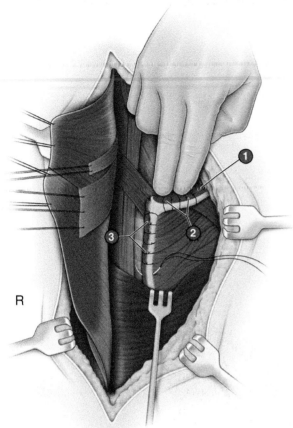

R

Sequence of muscle reattachments:

1. Supraspinatus to base of scapular spine

2. Subscapularis muscle to vertebral border

3. Serratus anterior to vertebral border
    at a level more proximal than
    its original position

Levator scapulae muscle
lengthened by Z-plasty

Muscle reattachments, cont'd:

4. Lengthened levator scapulae muscle to
    superior border of scapula

5. Rhomboids to medial border of scapula
    at more proximal site than original position

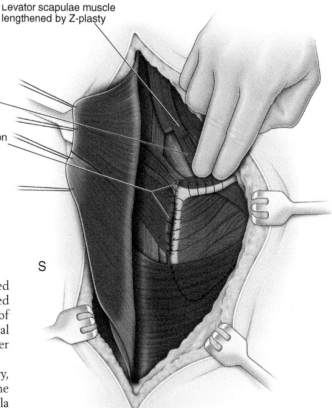

S

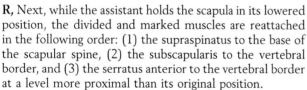

R, Next, while the assistant holds the scapula in its lowered position, the divided and marked muscles are reattached in the following order: (1) the supraspinatus to the base of the scapular spine, (2) the subscapularis to the vertebral border, and (3) the serratus anterior to the vertebral border at a level more proximal than its original position.
S, (4) The levator scapulae muscle, lengthened if necessary, is attached to the superior border of the scapula. (5) The rhomboids are attached to the medial border of the scapula at a more proximal site than the original position.

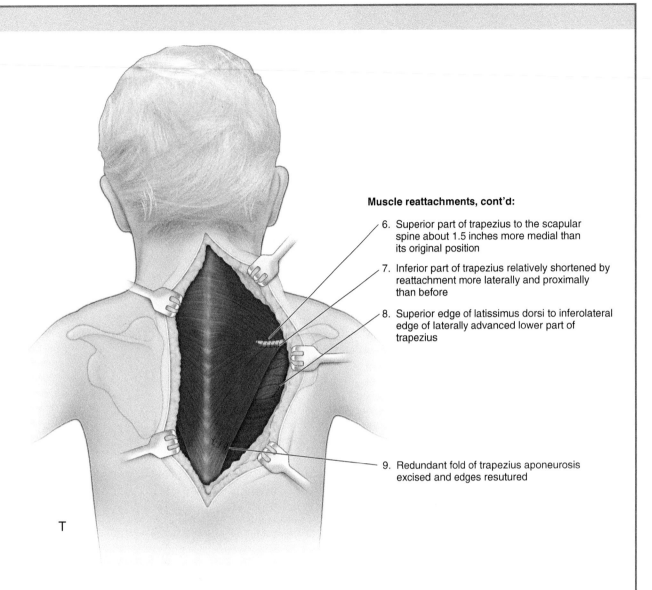

Muscle reattachments, cont'd:

6. Superior part of trapezius to the scapular spine about 1.5 inches more medial than its original position

7. Inferior part of trapezius relatively shortened by reattachment more laterally and proximally than before

8. Superior edge of latissimus dorsi to inferolateral edge of laterally advanced lower part of trapezius

9. Redundant fold of trapezius aponeurosis excised and edges resutured

T

T, (6) The superior part of the trapezius is reattached to the scapular spine about 1½ inches medial to its original position. (7) The inferior part of the trapezius is attached to the spine of the scapula more laterally and proximally than before. (8) The superior edge of the latissimus dorsi is attached to the inferolateral edge of the laterally advanced lower part of the trapezius. In the distal part of the incision, the origin of the lower part of the trapezius is followed, excess tissue is excised, and the free muscle edges are overlapped and sutured. The increased tension in this part of the muscle will serve as an added measure to hold the scapula in its lowered position. The wound is closed in layers. Closure of the skin should be subcuticular. If an associated pterygium colli is present, a Z-plasty repair may be performed.

Postoperative Care

The shoulder is immobilized in a Velpeau cast. Make sure that the elbow is not elevated. The patient is discharged from the hospital in 3 or 4 days. About 4 to 6 weeks postoperatively, the cast is removed and active shoulder abduction and scapular depression exercises are performed to increase muscle strength. Passive exercises of the glenohumeral and scapulocostal joints are carried out to increase range of joint motion.

Procedure 62   Woodward Operation for Congenital High Scapula

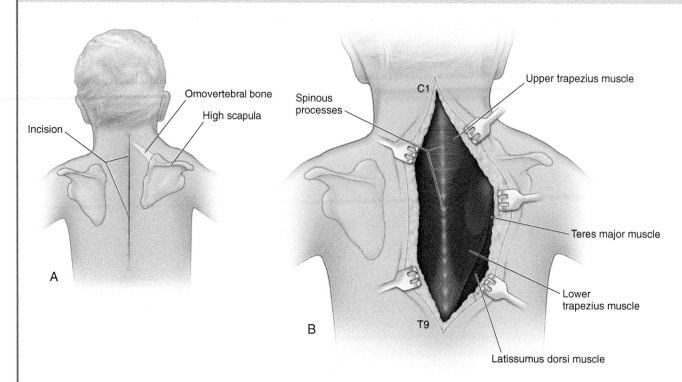

The operation is performed with the patient in the prone position, the head supported on a craniotomy headrest, and the neck in slight flexion. The sides and back of the neck, both shoulders, the trunk down to the iliac crests, and the upper limb on the involved side are prepared and draped. One should be able to manipulate the shoulder girdle and arms during the operation without contaminating the surgical field.

Operative Technique

A, A midline longitudinal incision is made that extends from the spinous process of the first cervical vertebra to that of the ninth thoracic vertebra.

B, The subcutaneous tissue is divided in line with the skin incision. The wound margins are undermined laterally to the medial border of the scapula. The muscle arrangement should be clearly visualized.

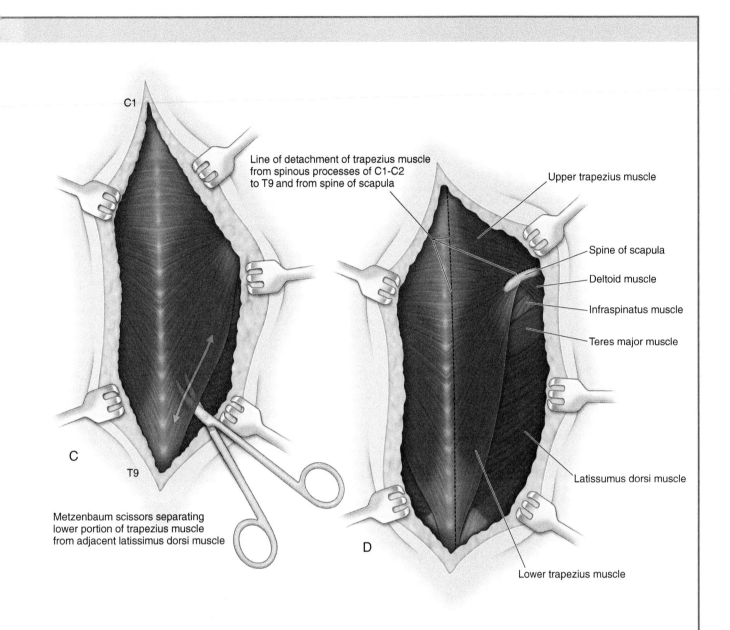

C, Next, the lateral border of the trapezius muscle is identified at the distal part of the wound. By blunt dissection, the lower portion of the trapezius is separated from the subjacent latissimus dorsi muscle.

D, With a sharp scalpel the tough and tendinous origin of the trapezius muscle is detached from the spinous process. Numerous sutures are passed at the entire origin of the muscle to mark it and for use at later reattachment.

Continued on following page

Procedure 62   Woodward Operation for Congenital High Scapula, cont'd

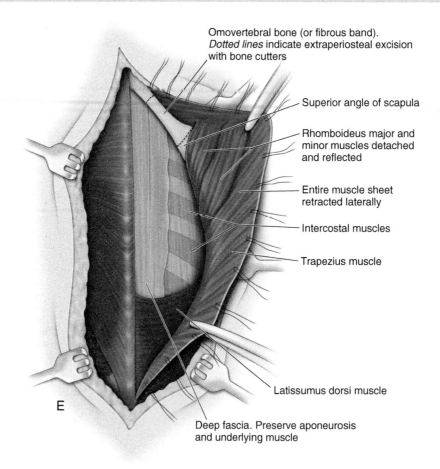

Omovertebral bone (or fibrous band).
Dotted lines indicate extraperiosteal excision
with bone cutters

Superior angle of scapula

Rhomboideus major and
minor muscles detached
and reflected

Entire muscle sheet
retracted laterally

Intercostal muscles

Trapezius muscle

Latissumus dorsi muscle

E

Deep fascia. Preserve aponeurosis
and underlying muscle

E, In the upper part of the incision the origins of the rhomboideus major and minor muscles are sharply divided and tagged with sutures. A well-defined deep layer of fascia separates the rhomboids and the upper part of the trapezius from the serratus posterior superior and erector spinae muscles. It is vital to maintain a proper tissue plane. Preserve the aponeurosis and muscle sheet intact for secure fixation of the scapula at its lowered level.

Next, the entire muscle sheet is retracted laterally to expose the omovertebral bone or fibrous band if present. The omovertebral bar is excised extraperiosteally; it usually extends from the superior angle of the scapula to the lower cervical vertebrae. It is best to use a bone cutter for resection. Avoid injury to the spinal accessory nerve, the nerves to the rhomboids, and the descending scapular artery. The contracted levator scapulae muscle is sectioned at its attachment to the scapula. Fibrous bands attached to the anterior surface of the scapula usually restrict its downward displacement; if present, they are sectioned. Next, the scapula is everted, and the serratus anterior muscle is detached from its insertion on the vertebral border of the scapula. A periosteal elevator is used to elevate the supraspinatus muscle extraperiosteally from the supraspinous portion of the scapula and the subscapularis muscle from the deep surface of the scapula midway between the superior and inferior angles. The supraspinous portion of the scapula is resected with its periosteum. The suprascapular vessels and nerves and the transverse scapular artery should be protected from injury. These steps are illustrated on Procedure 60, steps *K* and *L*, of the modified Green scapuloplasty.

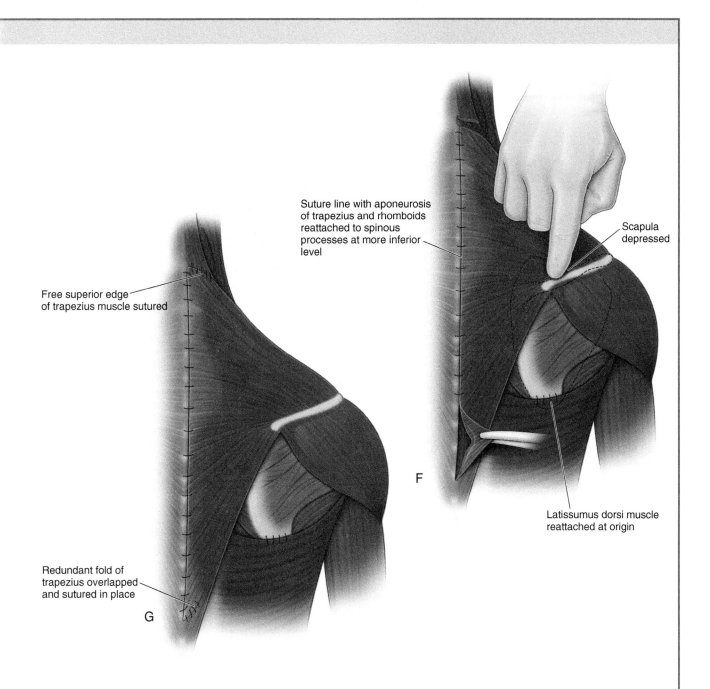

Suture line with aponeurosis of trapezius and rhomboids reattached to spinous processes at more inferior level

Scapula depressed

Free superior edge of trapezius muscle sutured

F

Latissumus dorsi muscle reattached at origin

Redundant fold of trapezius overlapped and sutured in place

G

F, Next, the scapula is lowered to its normal level and held in the corrected position by an assistant. The subscapularis muscle is reattached to the vertebral border of the scapula, and the supraspinatus muscle is resutured to the scapular spine. The serratus anterior muscle is reattached to the vertebral border of the scapula at a more proximal level. The latissimus dorsi muscle is reattached to the scapula. Proceeding cephalocaudally, the thick aponeurosis of the trapezius and rhomboid muscles is sutured to the spinous processes at a more distal level. It is essential that an assistant maintain the corrected level of the scapula.

G, Because the origin of the trapezius muscle distal to the ninth thoracic vertebra is not disturbed, a redundant fold

of aponeurotic tissue is created in the distal end of the trapezius muscle. This fold of soft tissue is excised and resutured.

The wound is closed in usual fashion. The skin closure is subcuticular.

Postoperative Care

A Velpeau bandage is applied and worn for 3 to 4 weeks. The patient is allowed to be up and around the day after the operation. After removal of the Velpeau bandage, postoperative exercises similar to those described for the modified Green scapuloplasty are carried out.

Procedure 63   Disarticulation of the Shoulder

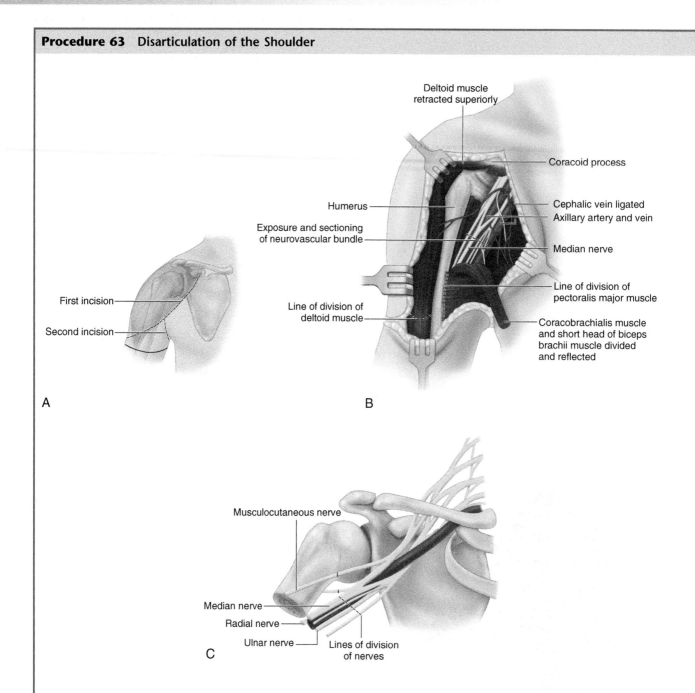

The patient is placed in a semilateral position so that the posterior aspect of the affected shoulder, scapula, and axilla and the entire upper limb can be prepared and draped in a sterile fashion.

A, The skin incision begins at the coracoid process and extends distally in the deltopectoral groove to the insertion of the deltoid muscle; it then continues proximally along the posterior border of the deltoid muscle to terminate at the posterior axillary fold. A second incision in the axilla connects the anterior and posterior borders of the first incision.

B, In the deltopectoral groove, the cephalic vein is identified, ligated, and transected. The deltoid muscle is retracted laterally to expose the humeral attachment of the pectoralis major muscle, which is divided at its

insertion and reflected medially. The coracobrachialis and short head of the biceps are divided at their origins from the coracoid process and reflected distally.

Next, the deltoid muscle is detached from its insertion on the humerus and retracted proximally.

C, The axillary artery and vein and the thoracoacromial vessels are identified, isolated, doubly ligated with size 0 silk sutures, and divided. The thoracoacromial artery is a short trunk branching from the anterior surface of the axillary artery. Its origin is usually covered by the pectoralis minor muscle. The median, ulnar, musculocutaneous, and radial nerves are identified, isolated, pulled distally, divided with a sharp knife, and allowed to retract beneath the pectoralis minor muscle.

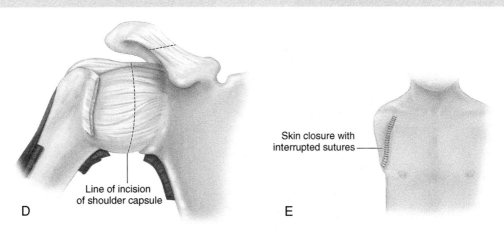

D

Line of incision
of shoulder capsule

E

Skin closure with
interrupted sutures

D, The capsule of the shoulder joint is exposed by retracting the deltoid muscle superiorly. Next, the arm is placed in marked external rotation. The subscapularis muscle, long head of the biceps at its origin, and anterior capsule of the shoulder joint are divided. The teres major and latissimus dorsi muscles are sectioned near their insertion to the intertubercular groove of the humerus. The acromion process is exposed extraperiosteally by elevating the origin of the deltoid muscle from its lateral border and superior surface. The acromion process is partially excised with an osteotome to give the shoulder a smooth, rounded contour.

The arm is placed across the chest, with the shoulder in marked internal rotation. The supraspinatus, infraspinatus, and teres minor muscles are divided at their insertion. The capsule of the shoulder joint is divided superiorly and posteriorly. The long head of the triceps brachii is sectioned near its origin from the infraglenoid tuberosity of the scapula. The inferior capsule of the joint is divided, completing disarticulation of the shoulder. The hyaline articular cartilage of the glenoid cavity is curetted, exposing cancellous, raw bleeding bone. The cut ends of the muscles are sutured to the glenoid fossa.

E, The deltoid muscle is sutured to the inferior aspect of the neck of the scapula. Suction catheters are placed deep to the deltoid muscle and connected to a suction evacuator. The subcutaneous tissue and skin are closed in layers with interrupted sutures.

Procedure 64   Amputation Through the Arm

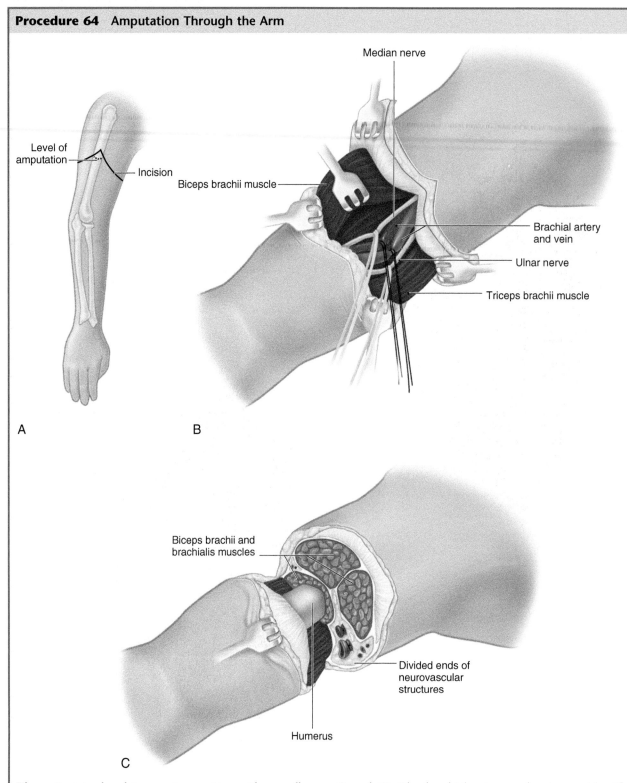

A

B

Median nerve

Biceps brachii muscle

Brachial artery
and vein

Ulnar nerve

Triceps brachii muscle

Biceps brachii and
brachialis muscles

Divided ends of
neurovascular
structures

Humerus

C

The patient is placed in a supine position with a sandbag under the shoulder that is to be operated on. A sterile tourniquet is applied in the axillary region for hemostasis.
A, Anterior and posterior skin flaps are fashioned so that they are equal in length and 1 cm longer than half the diameter of the arm at the intended level of amputation. The subcutaneous tissue and deep fascia are divided in line with the skin incision, and the wound flaps are retracted.

B and **C,** The brachial artery and vein are identified, doubly ligated, and divided. The median and ulnar nerves are isolated, pulled distally, sectioned with a sharp knife, and allowed to retract proximally. The muscles in the anterior compartment of the arm are divided 1.5 cm distal to the site of bone division, and the muscle mass is beveled distally.

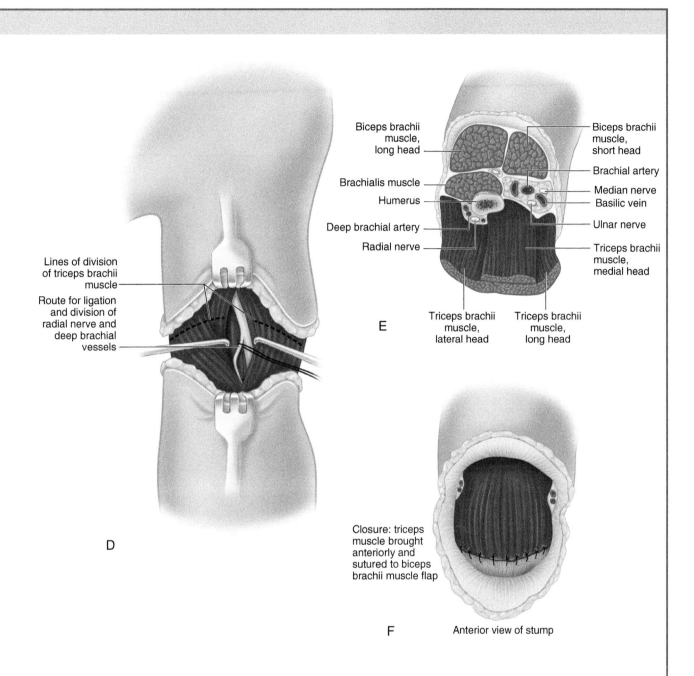

Lines of division of triceps brachii muscle

Route for ligation and division of radial nerve and deep brachial vessels

D

Biceps brachii muscle, long head

Brachialis muscle

Humerus

Deep brachial artery

Radial nerve

Biceps brachii muscle, short head

Brachial artery

Median nerve

Basilic vein

Ulnar nerve

Triceps brachii muscle, medial head

Triceps brachii muscle, lateral head

Triceps brachii muscle, long head

E

Closure: triceps muscle brought anteriorly and sutured to biceps brachii muscle flap

F   Anterior view of stump

D, The radial nerve is isolated, pulled distally, and sectioned with a sharp knife. The deep brachial vessels are doubly ligated and divided. The triceps brachii muscle is sectioned 3 to 4 cm distal to the level of the bone section and beveled to form a skin flap.

E, The humerus is divided, and the bone end is smoothed with a rasp.

F, The distal end of the triceps muscle is brought anteriorly and sutured to the deep fascia of the anterior compartment muscles. Catheters are inserted for closed suction, and the wound is closed with interrupted sutures.

Procedure 65   Disarticulation of the Elbow

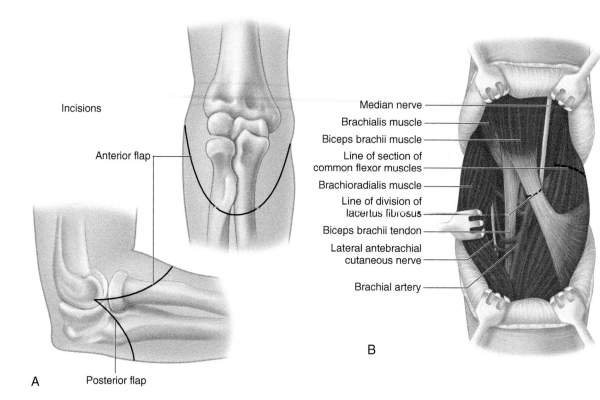

Incisions

Anterior flap

Posterior flap

A

Median nerve
Brachialis muscle
Biceps brachii muscle
Line of section of
common flexor muscles
Brachioradialis muscle
Line of division of
lacertus fibrosus
Biceps brachii tendon
Lateral antebrachial
cutaneous nerve
Brachial artery

B

The operation is performed with a pneumatic tourniquet on the proximal arm.

A, The anterior and posterior skin flaps are fashioned to be equal in length to the medial and lateral epicondyles of the humerus, which serve as the medial and lateral proximal points. The lower margin of the posterior flap is 2.5 cm distal to the tip of the olecranon; the distal margin of the anterior flap is immediately inferior to the insertion of the biceps tendon on the tuberosity of the radius.

B, The wound flaps are undermined and reflected 3 cm proximal to the level of the epicondyles of the humerus. The lacertus fibrosus is sectioned. The common flexor muscles of the forearm are divided at their origin from the medial epicondyle of the humerus, elevated extraperiosteally, and reflected distally.

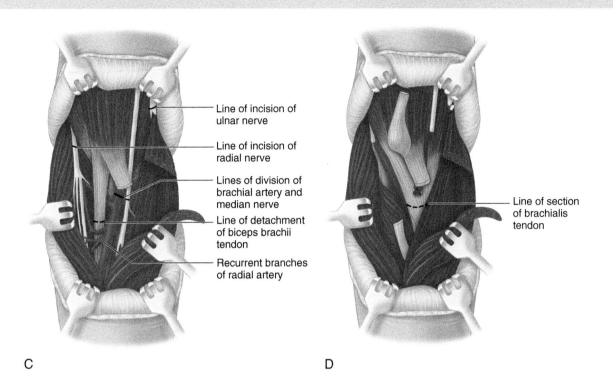

C

Line of incision of ulnar nerve

Line of incision of radial nerve

Lines of division of brachial artery and median nerve

Line of detachment of biceps brachii tendon

Recurrent branches of radial artery

D

Line of section of brachialis tendon

C and **D,** The brachial vessels and median nerve on the medial aspect of the biceps tendon are exposed. The brachial vessels are doubly ligated and divided proximal to the joint level. The median nerve is pulled distally, divided with a sharp knife, and allowed to retract proximally. The ulnar nerve is dissected free in its groove behind the medial epicondyle, drawn distally, and sharply sectioned. The biceps tendon is detached from its insertion on the radial tuberosity.

The radial nerve is isolated in the interval between the brachioradialis and brachialis muscles. The nerve is pulled distally and divided with a sharp knife. The brachialis muscle tendon is divided at its insertion to the coronoid process.

Continued on following page

Procedure 65   Disarticulation of the Elbow, cont'd

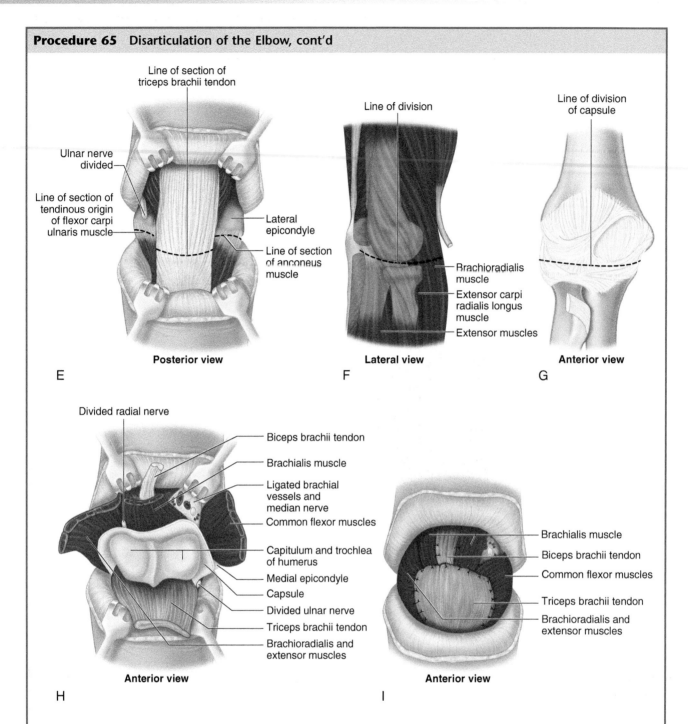

Line of section of
triceps brachii tendon

Ulnar nerve
divided

Line of section of
tendinous origin
of flexor carpi
ulnaris muscle

Lateral
epicondyle

Line of section
of anconeus
muscle

Posterior view

E

Line of division

Brachioradialis
muscle

Extensor carpi
radialis longus
muscle

Extensor muscles

Lateral view

F

Line of division
of capsule

Anterior view

G

Divided radial nerve

Biceps brachii tendon

Brachialis muscle

Ligated brachial
vessels and
median nerve

Common flexor muscles

Capitulum and trochlea
of humerus

Medial epicondyle

Capsule

Divided ulnar nerve

Triceps brachii tendon

Brachioradialis and
extensor muscles

Anterior view

H

Brachialis muscle

Biceps brachii tendon

Common flexor muscles

Triceps brachii tendon

Brachioradialis and
extensor muscles

Anterior view

I

E and **F,** The brachioradialis and common extensor muscles are sectioned transversely approximately 4 to 5 cm distal to the joint line. Following detachment of the triceps tendon at its insertion near the tip of the olecranon process, division of the common extensor muscles of the forearm is completed.

G and **H,** The capsule and ligaments of the elbow joint are divided, and the forearm is removed. The tourniquet is released, and complete hemostasis is obtained.

I, The triceps tendon is sutured to the brachialis and biceps tendons. The proximal segment of the extensor muscles of the forearm is brought laterally and sutured to the triceps tendon. The wound flaps are approximated with interrupted sutures. Catheters are placed in the wound for closed suction.

Procedure 66   Posterior Release of Elbow Extension Contracture

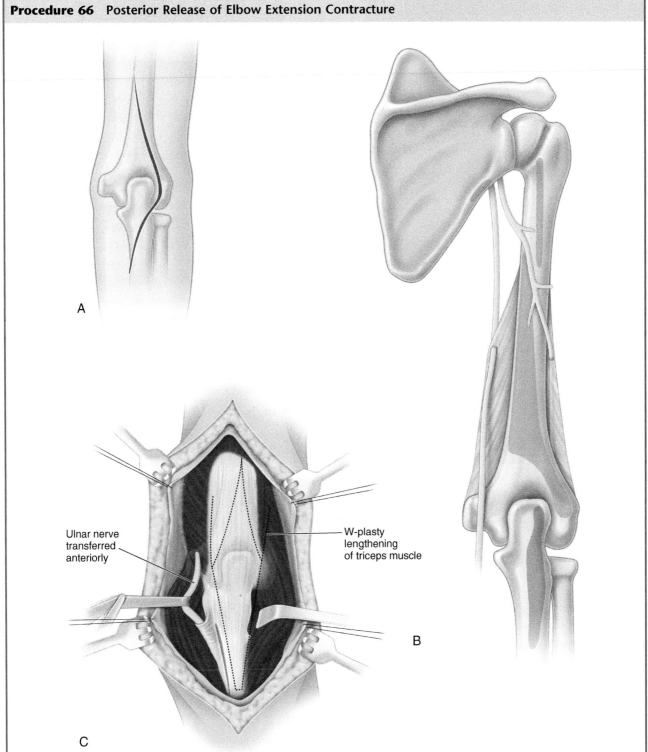

A

B

C

Ulnar nerve
transferred
anteriorly

W-plasty
lengthening
of triceps muscle

Operative Technique

A, The patient is placed in a lateral position. A midline incision is made on the posterior aspect of the arm, beginning in the middle half and extending distally to a point lateral to the olecranon process; the incision is then carried over the subcutaneous surface of the shaft of the ulna for a distance of 5 cm. The subcutaneous tissue is divided, and the wound flaps are mobilized.

B, The ulnar nerve is identified and mobilized medially to protect it from injury. The intermuscular septum is exposed laterally.
C, *Left,* The ulnar nerve is mobilized and transferred anteriorly. *Right,* The triceps muscle is lengthened in a W fashion, leaving a long proximal tongue.

Continued on following page

Procedure 66   Posterior Release of Elbow Extension Contracture, cont'd

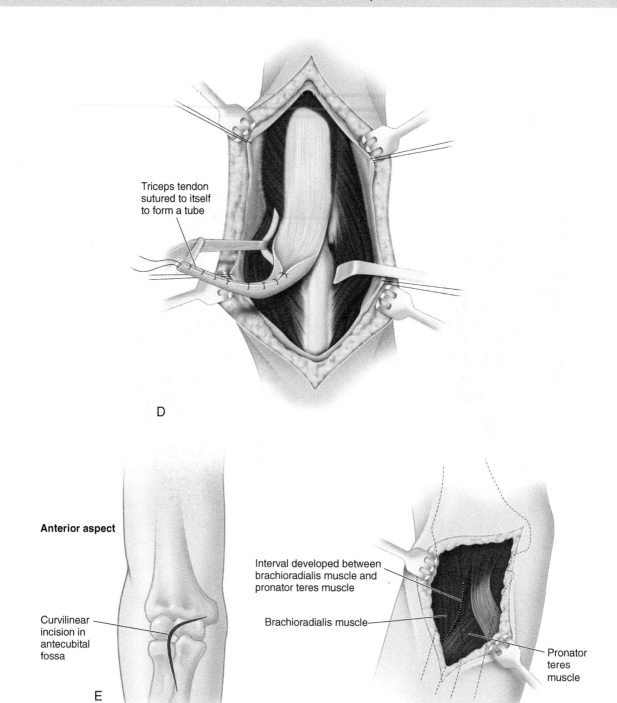

Triceps tendon sutured to itself to form a tube

D

Anterior aspect

Curvilinear incision in antecubital fossa

E

Interval developed between brachioradialis muscle and pronator teres muscle

Brachioradialis muscle

Pronator teres muscle

F

D, The triceps muscle is freed and mobilized proximally as far as its nerve supply permits. The motor branches of the radial nerve to the triceps enter the muscle in the interval between the lateral and medial heads as the radial nerve enters the musculospiral groove. The distal portion of the detached triceps is then sutured to itself to form a tube.

E and **F,** Through a curvilinear incision in the antecubital fossa, the interval between the brachioradialis and pronator teres is developed.

G, With an Ober tendon passer, the triceps tendon is passed into the anterior wound subcutaneously, superficial to the radial nerve.

H, With the elbow in 90 degrees of flexion and the forearm in full supination, the triceps tendon is sutured to the biceps tendon or anchored to the radial tuberosity by a suture passed through a drill hole. The wound is closed in a routine fashion. An above-elbow cast is applied, with the elbow in 90 degrees of flexion and full supination.

Postoperative Care

The cast is removed 4 weeks after surgery, and active exercises are performed to develop elbow flexion. Gravity provides extension to the elbow.

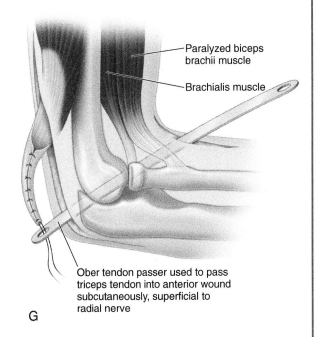

Paralyzed biceps brachii muscle

Brachialis muscle

Ober tendon passer used to pass triceps tendon into anterior wound subcutaneously, superficial to radial nerve

G

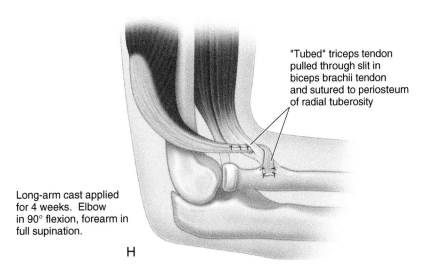

"Tubed" triceps tendon pulled through slit in biceps brachii tendon and sutured to periosteum of radial tuberosity

Long-arm cast applied for 4 weeks. Elbow in 90° flexion, forearm in full supination.

H

Procedure 67   **Posterior Approach for Forequarter Amputation (Littlewood Technique)**

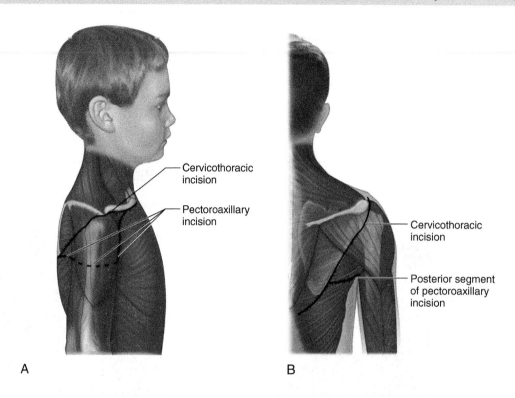

A   B

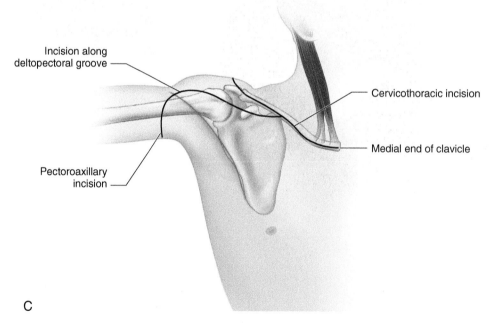

C

The patient is placed in the lateral position, and the neck, chest, and whole upper limb are prepared and draped. Blood loss is minimal, but adequate whole blood should be available for transfusion if necessary.

A to C, The cervicothoracic incision begins at the medial end of the clavicle and extends laterally along the antero-inferior border of the clavicle to the lateral protuberance of the acromion, where it curves posteriorly. It is then continued along the lateral border of the scapula to its inferior angle, where it curves medially to terminate 3 to 4 cm lateral to the midline of the spine.

The pectoroaxillary incision begins at the center of the clavicle and extends inferolaterally along the deltopectoral groove; it then crosses the anterior axillary fold and joins the posterior incision at the lower third of the lateral border of the scapula. The subcutaneous tissue and fascia are divided in line with the skin incision, and the wound flaps are mobilized to expose the underlying muscles.

D and **E,** The muscles connecting the scapula to the trunk are detached from the scapula in layers and marked with silk whip sutures. First, the trapezius and latissimus dorsi are divided.

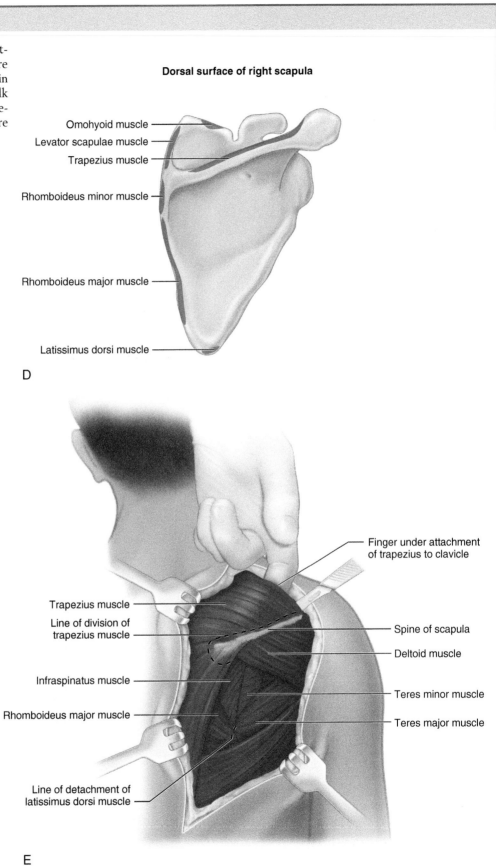

Dorsal surface of right scapula

Omohyoid muscle

Levator scapulae muscle

Trapezius muscle

Rhomboideus minor muscle

Rhomboideus major muscle

Latissimus dorsi muscle

D

Finger under attachment of trapezius to clavicle

Trapezius muscle

Line of division of trapezius muscle

Spine of scapula

Deltoid muscle

Infraspinatus muscle

Teres minor muscle

Rhomboideus major muscle

Teres major muscle

Line of detachment of latissimus dorsi muscle

E

Continued on following page

Procedure 67   **Posterior Approach for Forequarter Amputation (Littlewood Technique), cont'd**

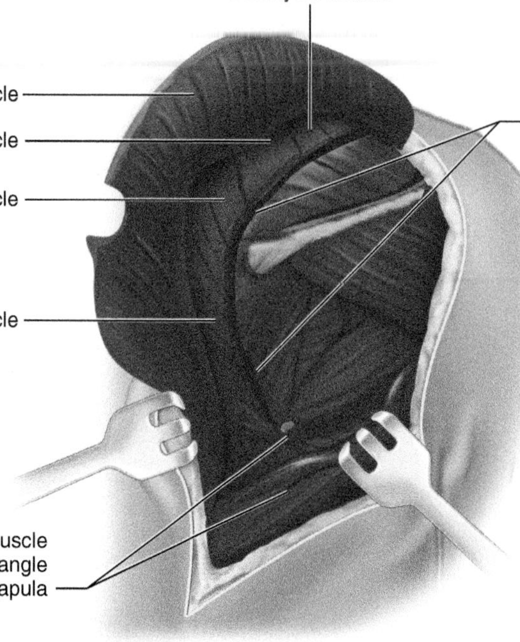

Omohyoid muscle

Trapezius muscle

Levator scapulae muscle

Rhomboideus minor muscle

Rhomboideus major muscle

Division of omohyoid, levator scapulae, and rhomboid muscles

Latissimus dorsi muscle detached at inferior angle of scapula

F

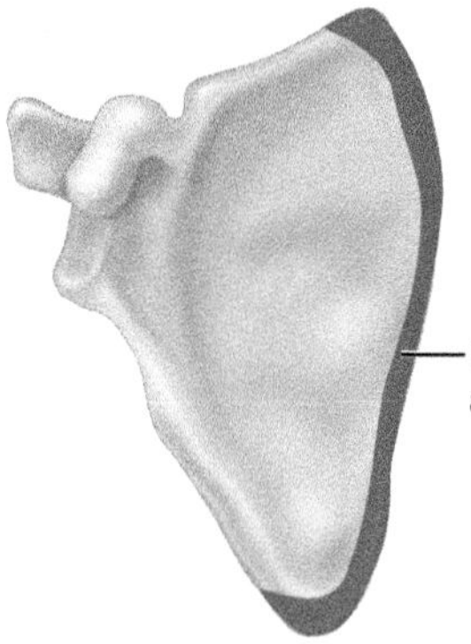

Insertion of serratus anterior muscle

Scapula retracted

Divided portion of serratus anterior muscle

Scalpel dividing serratus anterior muscle

G

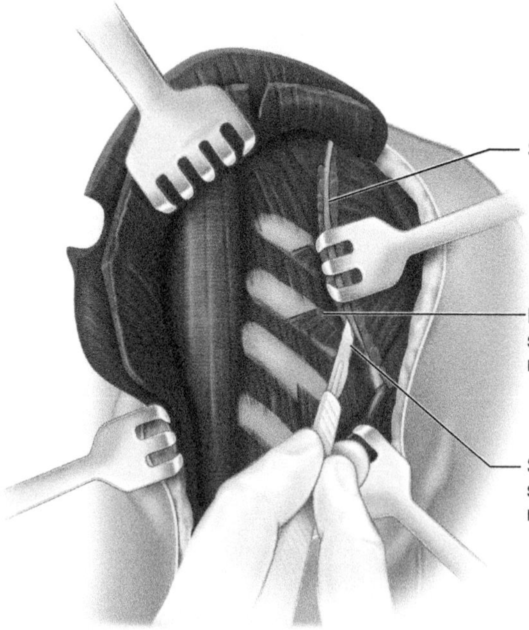

H

F, Next, the omohyoid, levator scapulae, and rhomboid muscles are detached. Transverse cervical and transverse scapular vessels are ligated and divided as dissection proceeds. The cords of the brachial plexus are sectioned with a very sharp scalpel near their origin.

G and H, The scapula is retracted forward, and the serratus anterior muscle is sectioned and detached from the scapula.

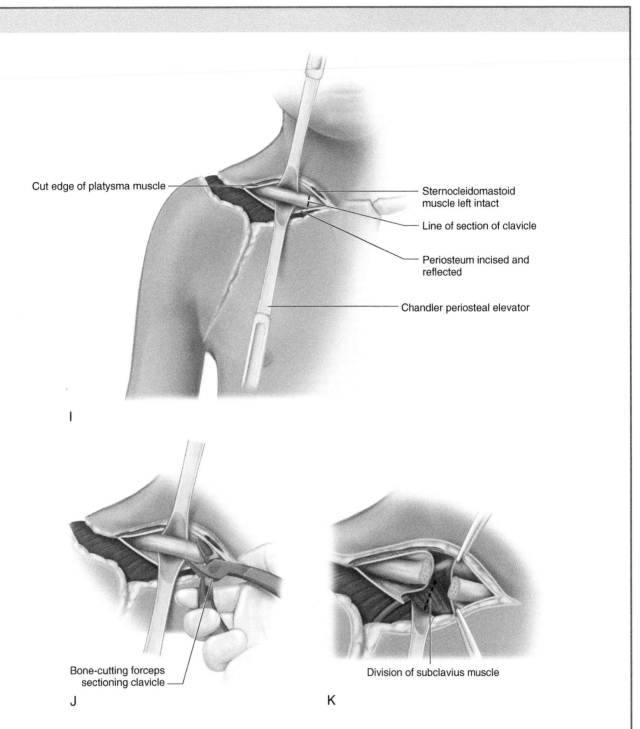

Cut edge of platysma muscle

Sternocleidomastoid muscle left intact

Line of section of clavicle

Periosteum incised and reflected

Chandler periosteal elevator

I

Bone-cutting forceps sectioning clavicle

J

Division of subclavius muscle

K

I to K, The patient is turned onto her or his back, and the medial end of the clavicle is exposed subperiosteally. Lever-type retractors are placed deep to the clavicle to protect the underlying neurovascular structures. With bone-cutting forceps or a Gigli saw, the clavicle is sectioned near its sternal attachment. The subclavius muscle is divided next.

Continued on following page

Procedure 67   **Posterior Approach for Forequarter Amputation (Littlewood Technique), cont'd**

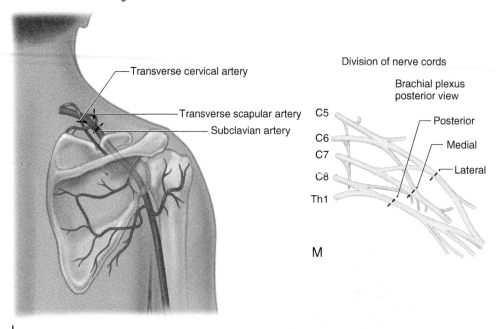

Ligation and division of arteries

Transverse cervical artery

Transverse scapular artery

Subclavian artery

Division of nerve cords

Brachial plexus
posterior view

C5

C6

C7

C8

Th1

Posterior

Medial

Lateral

M

L

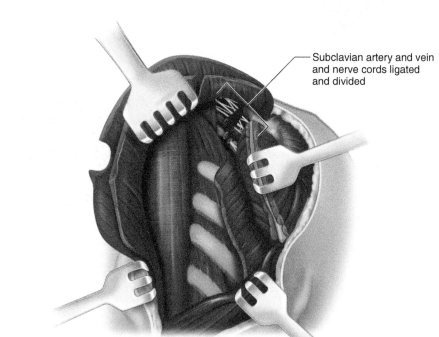

Subclavian artery and vein
and nerve cords ligated
and divided

N

L to **N,** The subclavian vessels and brachial plexus are exposed by allowing the upper limb to fall anteriorly. The subclavian artery and vein are isolated, individually clamped, doubly ligated with sutures, and divided.

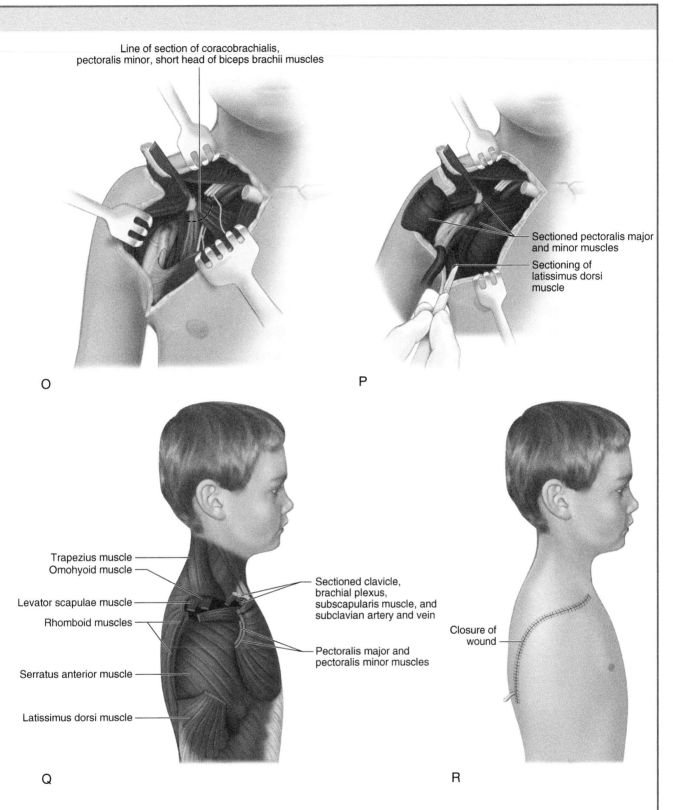

Line of section of coracobrachialis,
pectoralis minor, short head of biceps brachii muscles

Sectioned pectoralis major
and minor muscles

Sectioning of
latissimus dorsi
muscle

O

P

Trapezius muscle
Omohyoid muscle

Levator scapulae muscle

Rhomboid muscles

Serratus anterior muscle

Latissimus dorsi muscle

Sectioned clavicle,
brachial plexus,
subscapularis muscle, and
subclavian artery and vein

Pectoralis major and
pectoralis minor muscles

Closure of
wound

Q

R

O to Q, The pectoralis major and minor, short head of the biceps, coracobrachialis, and latissimus dorsi are sectioned, completing ablation of the limb.

R, The wound flaps are approximated and sutured together. Closed suction catheters are inserted and connected to an evacuator. A firm compression dressing is applied.

Procedure 68   **Flexorplasty of the Elbow (the Mayer and Green Modification of the Steindler Technique)**

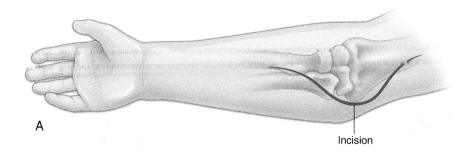

A

Incision

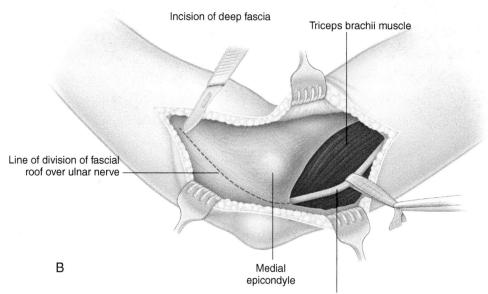

Incision of deep fascia

Triceps brachii muscle

Line of division of fascial
roof over ulnar nerve

B

Medial
epicondyle

Ulnar nerve retracted

Operative Technique

A, With the elbow in extension, a curved longitudinal incision is made over the anteromedial side of the elbow, beginning approximately 3 in above the flexion crease of the elbow joint over the medial intermuscular septum and extending distally to the anterior aspect of the medial epicondyle. At the joint level it turns anterolaterally on the volar surface of the forearm along the course of the pronator teres muscle for a distance of approximately 2 in.

B, The subcutaneous tissue and fascia are divided in line with the skin incision, and the skin flaps are widely mobilized and retracted. Next the ulnar nerve is located posterior to the medial intermuscular septum and lying in a groove on the triceps muscle. It is isolated, and moist hernia tape is passed around it for gentle handling. The ulnar nerve is traced distally to its groove between the posterior aspect of the medial epicondyle of the humerus and the olecranon process. The fascial roof over the ulnar nerve is carefully divided under direct vision over a grooved director.

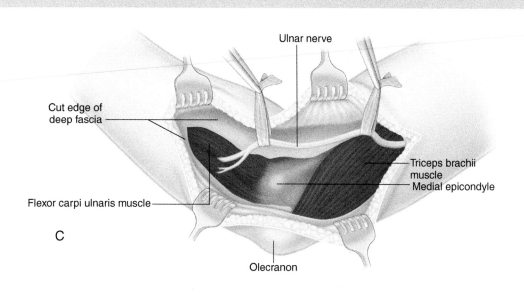

C

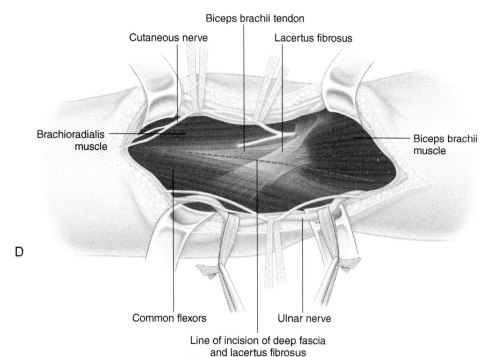

D

C, The ulnar nerve is dissected free distally to the point where it passes between the two heads of the flexor carpi ulnaris muscle. Inadvertent damage to branches of the ulnar nerve to the flexor carpi ulnaris should be avoided. A second piece of hernia tape is passed around the ulnar nerve in the distal part of the wound, and the nerve is retracted posteriorly.

D, Next the biceps tendon is identified over the anterior aspect of the elbow joint. The deep fascia and the lacertus fibrosus are divided along the medial aspect of the biceps tendon.

Continued on following page

Procedure 68   **Flexorplasty of the Elbow (the Mayer and Green Modification of the Steindler Technique), cont'd**

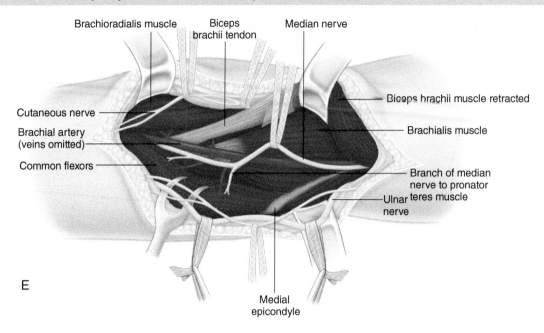

E

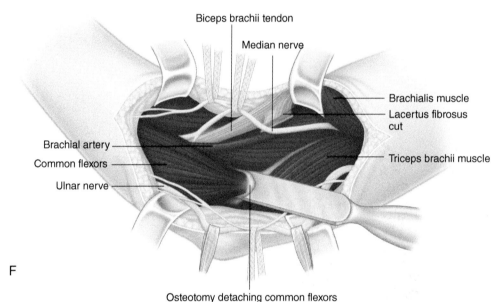

F

E, By digital palpation, the interval between the biceps and pronator teres muscle is developed. The brachial artery with its accompanying veins runs along the medial side of the biceps tendon. The median nerve, lying medial to the brachial artery, is dissected free of surrounding tissue and gently retracted anteriorly with moist hernia tape. The branches of the median nerve to the pronator teres muscle must be identified and protected from injury.

F, Next, with an osteotome, the common flexor origin of the pronator teres, the flexor carpi radialis, the palmaris longus, the flexor digitorum sublimis, and the flexor carpi ulnaris is detached en bloc with a flake of bone from the medial epicondyle.

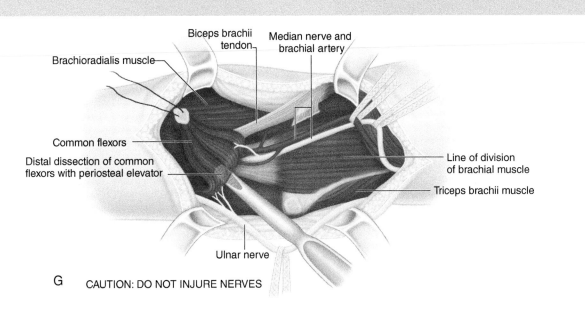

G   CAUTION: DO NOT INJURE NERVES

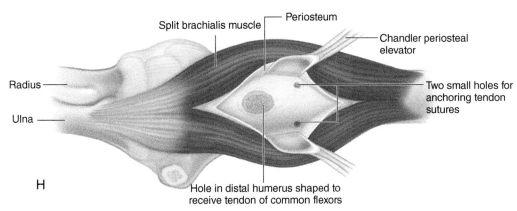

H

G, By sharp and blunt dissection, the flexor muscle mass is freed and mobilized distally away from the joint capsule and the ulna as far as the motor branches of the median nerve and ulnar nerve will permit. A no. 1 silk whip suture is placed in the proximal end of the common flexors.

H, The biceps muscle, brachial vessels, and median nerve are retracted laterally, and the atrophied brachial muscle is split longitudinally. The periosteum is incised and stripped to expose the anterior aspect of the distal end of the humerus.

The elbow is then flexed to 120 degrees to determine the site of attachment of the transfer (usually 2 in proximal to the elbow). With a drill, a hole is made on the anterior surface of the humerus. The opening is enlarged with progressively larger diamond-head hand drills to receive the transferred muscle. The action of the transfer as a pronator of the forearm is decreased by transferring it laterally on the humerus. With smaller drill points, two tunnels are made from the lateral and medial cortices of the humerus and connected to the larger hole for passing the suture.

Continued on following page

Procedure 68   Flexorplasty of the Elbow (the Mayer and Green Modification of the Steindler Technique), cont'd

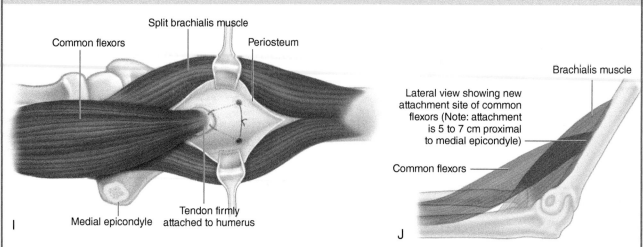

I — Common flexors — Split brachialis muscle — Periosteum — Medial epicondyle — Tendon firmly attached to humerus

J — Lateral view showing new attachment site of common flexors (Note: attachment is 5 to 7 cm proximal to medial epicondyle) — Common flexors — Brachialis muscle

I and **J,** Because the elbow will be immobilized in acute flexion, it is best to close the distal half of the wound before anchoring the transplant to the humerus. The ends of the whip suture are brought out through the tunnels, and the common flexors and the origin are firmly secured in the larger hole. The periosteum is closed with interrupted sutures over the transferred tendon, thus reinforcing its anchorage. The proximal half of the wound is closed, and a long-arm cast is applied with the elbow in acute flexion and the forearm in full supination.

For postoperative care, see the guidelines outlined in the text on principles of tendon transfer.

Procedure 69   Pectoralis Major Transfer for Paralysis of the Elbow Flexors

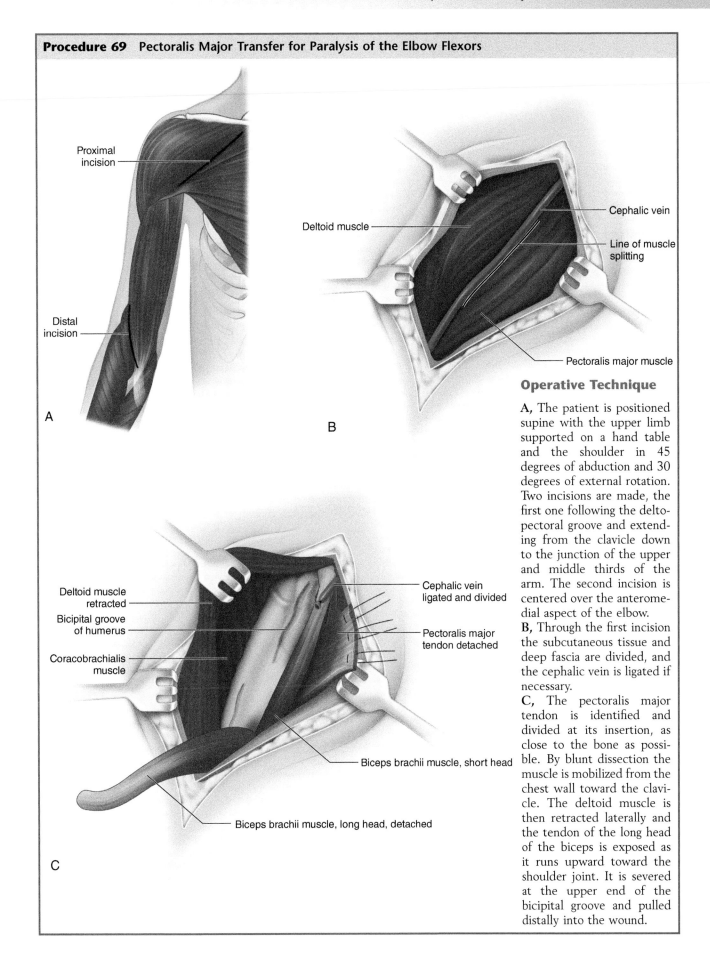

Proximal incision

Distal incision

A

Deltoid muscle

Cephalic vein

Line of muscle splitting

Pectoralis major muscle

B

Deltoid muscle retracted

Bicipital groove of humerus

Coracobrachialis muscle

Cephalic vein ligated and divided

Pectoralis major tendon detached

Biceps brachii muscle, short head

Biceps brachii muscle, long head, detached

C

Operative Technique

A, The patient is positioned supine with the upper limb supported on a hand table and the shoulder in 45 degrees of abduction and 30 degrees of external rotation. Two incisions are made, the first one following the delto-pectoral groove and extending from the clavicle down to the junction of the upper and middle thirds of the arm. The second incision is centered over the anterome-dial aspect of the elbow.

B, Through the first incision the subcutaneous tissue and deep fascia are divided, and the cephalic vein is ligated if necessary.

C, The pectoralis major tendon is identified and divided at its insertion, as close to the bone as possible. By blunt dissection the muscle is mobilized from the chest wall toward the clavicle. The deltoid muscle is then retracted laterally and the tendon of the long head of the biceps is exposed as it runs upward toward the shoulder joint. It is severed at the upper end of the bicipital groove and pulled distally into the wound.

Procedure 69   Pectoralis Major Transfer for Paralysis of the Elbow Flexors, cont'd

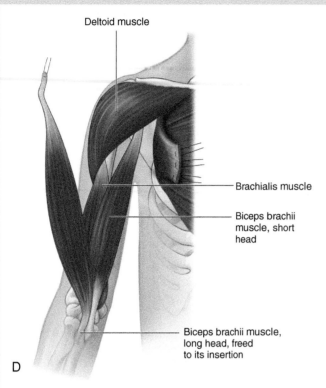

Deltoid muscle

Brachialis muscle

Biceps brachii muscle, short head

Biceps brachii muscle, long head, freed to its insertion

D

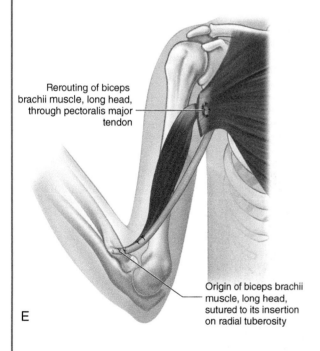

Rerouting of biceps brachii muscle, long head, through pectoralis major tendon

Origin of biceps brachii muscle, long head, sutured to its insertion on radial tuberosity

E

D, By blunt and sharp dissection, the muscle belly of the long head of the biceps is mobilized to the lowest third of the arm by freeing it from the short head. The vessels and nerves entering the muscle belly are divided and ligated as necessary. The tendon and muscle of the long head are delivered into the distal second incision and freed down to the tuberosity of the radius. Often, freeing the muscle from adhesions to the overlying fascia requires sharp dissection. After complete mobilization of the long head of the biceps by traction on its proximal end, the operator should be able to flex the elbow.

E, The long head of the biceps is pulled into the upper wound. Two slits are made in the tendon of the mobilized pectoralis major through which the tendon of the long head is passed, looped on itself, and brought down again into the distal wound. With the elbow acutely flexed, the proximal end of the tendon is sutured to its own tendon of insertion through a slit in the distal part of the tendon. Silk sutures are also inserted at the level of the tendon of the pectoralis major. The incisions are then closed in routine manner. A plaster-of-Paris–reinforced Velpeau bandage is applied with the elbow acutely flexed.

Postoperative Care

Plaster-of-Paris immobilization is continued for 3 weeks. At the end of this time active flexion and extension exercises of the elbow are started, first with gravity eliminated and then against gravity. A sling is used to protect the transferred tendon from stretching. Care should be taken to extend the elbow gradually so that active flexion above the right-angle position is maintained. Extension of the elbow is regained slowly.

INDEX

Note: Page numbers followed by "*f*" refer to illustrations; page numbers followed by "*t*" refer to tables; page numbers followed by "*b*" refer to boxes.